**REHABILITATION OF ATHLETIC INJURIES:
AN ATLAS OF THERAPEUTIC EXERCISE**

Rehabilitation of Athletic Injuries: An Atlas of Therapeutic Exercise

JOSEPH S. TORG, M.D.
Professor of Orthopaedic Surgery
Director, Sports Medicine Center
University of Pennsylvania
Philadelphia, Pennsylvania

JOSEPH J. VEGSO, M.S., A.T.C.
Head Athletic Trainer
Sports Medicine Center
University of Pennsylvania
Philadelphia, Pennsylvania

ELISABETH TORG, B.A.
Research Associate
Sports Medicine Center
University of Pennsylvania
Philadelphia, Pennsylvania

YEAR BOOK MEDICAL PUBLISHERS, INC.

Chicago • London • Boca Raton • Littleton, Mass.

5 6 7 8 9 0 CY 91 90

Library of Congress Cataloging-in-Publication Data

Torg, Joseph S.
   Rehabilitation of athletic injuries.

   Includes bibliographies and index.
   1. Sports—Accidents and injuries—Treatment.
2. Wounds and injuries—Patients—Rehabilitation.
I. Vegso, Joseph J. II. Torg, Elisabeth. III. Title.
[DNLM: 1. Athletic Injuries—diagnosis. 2. Athletic
Injuries—rehabilitation. QT 260 T682r]
RD97.T67 1987   617′.1027   86-26731
ISBN 0-8151-8820-X

Sponsoring Editor: Richard H. Lampert

Assistant Manager, Copyediting Services: Deborah Thorp

Production Project Manager: Max Perez

Proofroom Supervisor: Shirley E. Taylor

This book is dedicated to our gals, Olde Mom and Jude.

Preface

Proprioceptive neuromuscular facilitation . . . electrogalvanic stimulation . . . isokinetic dynamometry . . . therapeutic exercise regimen: the new talk of the 1980s. Sports medicine is in and therapeutic exercise is where it's at.

A redefinition of the term "the athlete" has recently occurred. A mere 20 years ago this designation required being a participating member of the varsity "nine," varsity "five," or varsity "eleven." Today most everyone considers himself an "athlete," and it is the rare individual who is not exhausting his or her bodily systems in the pursuit of the pleasures and the presumed benefits that physical activity bestows in the form of improved health and well-being. Preadolescents participate in Little League, midget league, pony league, and Pop Warner League activities. Adolescent participation in sports and games usually involves the school or neighborhood recreational teams. The most explosive involvement in physical activity, however, has been in the young adult and middle-aged populations. Literally millions in our society run half-marathons and marathons, participate in triathlons, ski, play tennis, ride bicycles, etc. As a people, we are on the move. Americans have awakened from their lethargy, gotten off their sedentary duffs, and—in many instances—are destroying themselves in the pursuit of physical fitness. It is for the "American Athlete" that this volume is intended.

The sports medicine surgeon is dedicated to the proposition that "to cut is to cure." The entrepreneurial cadre that has emerged recently to sell "sports" lotions, potions, shoes, suits, and sundry other devices is dedicated to the concept that healing can be merchandised at the local dry-goods store. We are committed to the concept that for the greatest number, the resolution of most athletic injuries is ensured by the appropriate implementation of rehabilitative and therapeutic exercise.

Although the sale of lotions, potions, gimmicks, and gadgets, as well as the performance of such sophisticated medical procedures as arthroscopic surgery certainly contribute to the well-being of the local—if not national—economy, most athletic injury problems will be responsive to the application of the appropriate balance of heat and cold, rest and exercise. Specifically, in the acute phase of most athletic injuries, a combination of rest and cold is effective. The use of heat and exercise is appropriate in the subacute phase. We have attempted, throughout this volume, to provide guidelines regarding management

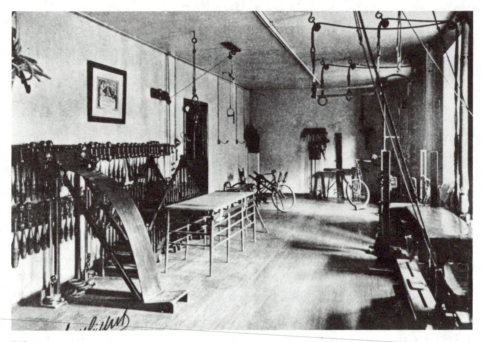

FIG 1.
The Hospital of the University of Pennsylvania orthopedic gymnasium circa 1900. (Courtesy of the archive of the University of Pennsylvania.)

of the characteristic and prototypical injuries commonly seen in an active sports medicine clinic. As indicated, these guidelines involve balancing heat and cold, rest and exercise, and—in those instances where indicated—use of pharmacologic agents. Also, when indicated, the currently recognized supportive and orthotic devices are described.

Although the nature of the athletes, their injuries, and the therapeutic and surgical modalities have changed over the years, the basic principles of therapeutic exercise have, for the most part, remained constant. The exercise devices in use at the turn of this century are antiquated in appearance. However, they represent the tools of the early therapist to implement functional rehabilitation through programs that increase joint motion, muscular strength, and cardiovascular aerobic capacity (Fig 1). The high-tech machines and devices of today, making up the mystique of the sports medicine center, in reality do little more (Fig 2). That is, they are designed to increase muscle strength, increase joint motion, and improve cardiovascular aerobic capacity. In the following pages we will attempt to impart to the reader simple, basic, and relatively unsophisticated principles that are the foundation of programs intended to rehabilitate the injured and postsurgical athlete. The emphasis of this volume will primarily involve the principles of therapeutic exercise.

JOSEPH S. TORG, M.D.
JOSEPH J. VEGSO, M.S., A.T.C.
ELISABETH TORG, B.A.

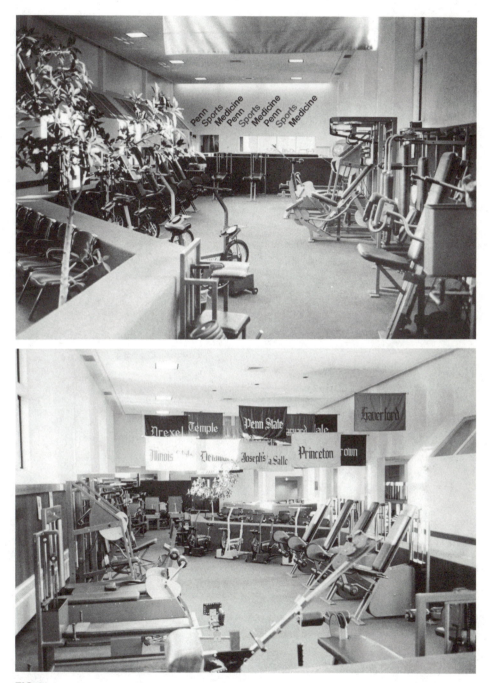

FIG 2.
University of Pennsylvania Sports Medicine Center—1986.

Contents

CHAPTER 1

Modalities

In rehabilitating the injured athlete, emphasis must be placed on an appropriate and well-supervised exercise program designed to restore range of motion, flexibility, strength, cardiovascular endurance, and agility. Without this emphasis the athlete will not be able to return to activity safely or at an effective level of performance.

Throughout this book, the importance of aggressive rehabilitation is clearly evident. The physician, athletic trainer, or physical therapist can utilize modalities as they deem necessary to supplement the rehabilitation programs that are provided.

THERAPEUTIC EXERCISE

In today's fast-paced, fitness-conscious society, the concept of therapeutic exercise has become diluted to the point that the majority of active Americans believe that any and all exercise is therapeutic. From the perspective of the athletic injury and rehabilitation, this belief could not be further from the truth.

The concept of therapeutic exercise falls under the domain of rehabilitation. To provide an injured athlete with a rehabilitation program that allows a safe and effective return to activity, a variety of factors must be taken into consideration. These factors include both the athlete's and physician's ultimate expectations for return to activity, the total disability of the athlete, and all of the parameters of physical fitness. Keeping the total well-being of the injured athlete in perspective is a significant factor in providing and maintaining a good professional relationship.

Much material has been written about rehabilitation, therapeutic exercise, and therapeutic modalities. Very little, however, has been directed specifically to the injured athlete. Because of this, there is a misconception that rehabilitation of the injured athlete must involve a staggering array of exercise and electronic equipment.

If the physician maintains the philosophy that rehabilitation of the athlete should be directed toward regaining range of motion, flexibility, strength, cardiorespiratory endurance, agility, and coordination, most athletes will be able to return to activity. However, if the physician simply provides analgesics and therapeutic modalities to treat the athlete's symptoms, i.e., pain, swelling, and stiffness, the athlete will not be able to return to activity safely or effectively.

Therefore, our goal throughout the text, and specifically in this chapter, is to provide the reader with an approach to rehabilitation that emphasizes therapeutic exercise.

FLEXIBILITY: RANGE OF MOTION

Range of motion and flexibility are usually considered to be synonymous. However, by definition there are subtle differences.

Range of motion refers to the movement of a specific joint. This motion is influenced by several structures: bony congruence, the joint capsule, ligamentous structures, and the muscles and tendons acting on the joint. Injury, surgery, or immobilization may affect one or more of these structures, thereby reducing or totally restricting range of motion.

Flexibility most frequently refers to the ability of a muscle to elongate as a joint or body segment moves through a range of motion. The same factors that can adversely affect joint range of motion may also reduce muscle flexibility.

The first step in the rehabilitation process is to initiate a set of exercises to increase range of motion and flexibility. There are several methods of stretching a joint and muscle to increase motion. The simplest and most effective is a slow, steady stretch that places the joint and/or muscle in the extreme range of available motion. This position is then maintained between 10 to 30 seconds or more, depending on patient tolerance. It can be done actively or passively. The amount of force used to stretch the joint or muscle is dependent on several factors: length of time since injury or surgery, the severity of injury, the surgical procedure, the joint involved, length of immobilization, and patient tolerance.

Range of motion exercises may be preceded with application of moist heat via whirlpools, hydrocollator steam packs, or warm showers when the injury is past the inflammatory stage.[7]

The general guidelines for static stretching and range of motion are as follows:

- The athlete must be relaxed.
- The motion or stretch position must be entered slowly.
- The stretch should produce a comfortable sensation.
- The stretch position should be maintained for 10 to 30 seconds and repeated ten or more times.

PROPRIOCEPTIVE NEUROMUSCULAR FACILITATION

Proprioceptive neuromuscular facilitation, or PNF, is a method employed to regain range of motion, flexibility, and neuromuscular function. The theory of PNF is based on stimulation of the proprioceptors, the Golgi tendon organs, and nerve endings. The athlete executes functional movement patterns, which begin with the muscles to be facilitated at a maximally stretched position and end with muscles at the maximally shortened end of their range.[1] A variety of simple and complex motor patterns are used to invoke improvements in motion, strength, and functional responses to stress placed on the muscles and joints. Proprioceptive neuromuscular facilitation can be achieved through numerous techniques which require substantial knowledge and skill.[4, 6] It is recommended that these techniques be learned before they are utilized in a rehabilitation setting.

STRENGTH

Muscular strength is an extremely important factor in athletic performance. Following injury or surgery, a significant portion of the rehabilitation program must be devoted to regaining strength in the muscle groups that have been injured or immobilized. In addition, one must not lose sight of the loss of strength in the other muscle groups that aid in supporting and stabilizing the injured joint, or those muscles that are affected by simple disuse.

In recent years there has been a tremendous growth in the variety of devices available for strengthening muscles. Despite the overabundance of equipment, the basic principles of strengthening muscle have remained unchanged. The following review of terminology and techniques is coupled with recommendations for applying these techniques to a rehabilitation program.

Muscle strength is defined as the maximum force that a muscle can exert in a single maximum contraction. Strength can be further defined as being static or dynamic. Static strength is commonly associated with a muscular contraction without joint movement (i.e., isometric), whereas dynamic strength involves a contraction with associated joint movement. Furthermore, a muscular contraction can be concentric or eccentric in nature. Concentric muscular contraction occurs when a muscle is contracted against resistance and the muscle shortens in length. Eccentric muscular contraction refers to a contraction of a muscle against a resistance while the muscle lengthens (i.e., the biceps muscle goes through an eccentric contraction as one lowers a dumbbell after doing a biceps curl).

An important aspect of the eccentric contraction is that a muscle can produce more force during this phase than during the concentric phase. This has implications during the rehabilitation program if an athlete cannot produce enough force to complete a concentric workout. Eccentric contraction workouts can be used effectively to increase strength in the early phases of rehabilitation. Methods of strengthening muscles fall into three main areas: isometric, isotonic, and isokinetic.

ISOMETRIC EXERCISE

Isometric exercise is typically defined as being a muscular contraction without associated movement of the joint or limb on which the muscle or muscles act.

Simply put, the force a muscle generates is less than or equal to the resistance being applied. The effectiveness of isometric exercise in increasing strength first gained notoriety in the 1950s as a result of the work of Hettinger and Muller.[2] The most recognizable and popular technique of exercising a muscle is to contract the muscle for 6 seconds at two-thirds maximum effort. The number of repetitions can be varied depending on the phase of rehabilitation and muscle condition.

There are several implications for the use of isometric strengthening exercises in a rehabilitation setting. Isometric strengthening is most effective in the very early stages of rehabilitation when joint motion is limited or not advisable, when the force that a muscle produces is not sufficient to utilize weights or other resistance equipment, and in athletes or patients who have conditions that do not allow for strengthening through an isotonic method.

Isometric exercise is convenient because it requires minimal equipment and supervision.

ISOTONIC EXERCISE

Isotonic exercise is defined as a strengthening exercise in which the muscle length shortens and a joint moves through a range of motion against a constant resistance or weight. This is easily accomplished through the use of a barbell, sandbag, weight bench, or other more sophisticated equipment such as an N-K table or Universal gym.

As the weight is lifted the muscle fatigues. Ideally a weight (resistance) is selected that causes the muscle to fatigue with a maximum of 6–10 repetitions. Over time, the muscle adapts and increases in strength. When this occurs it becomes easier to lift the weight. Additional weight is added to overload the muscle(s). This cycle is referred to as progressive resistance exercise, or PRE. Developed by De Lorme in the 1940s, it is the hallmark of muscle-strengthening programs. Since that time, many variations on the theory have been introduced. The basic principle remains unchanged. The amount of weight that is lifted must be increased progressively in order to increase muscle strength.

Typically, a minimum of three sets of six to ten repetitions of each exercise are performed during each rehabilitation session. In many instances, the injured athlete can perform strength exercises every day.

When isotonic exercises are used for rehabilitation it is important to monitor the patient on a regular basis, daily if possible, to be sure that the exercise program is not aggravating the injury. Swelling, discomfort, pain, effusion, and loss of motion are important warning signs that indicate the athlete is not ready for an isotonic strengthening program or that he or she is progressing too rapidly.

VARIABLE RESISTANCE

A variation of the isotonic strengthening method that has become popular in recent years is variable resistance exercise. Simply stated, like isotonics, the joints or muscle groups move through a range of motion against resistance. Unlike isotonics, however, the resistance varies to mimic or reproduce the mechanical advantages of the muscle and joint so that the muscle must work at a near maximum force throughout the range of motion.

Common examples of variable resistance equipment are: Nautilus, Universal-DVR, and CAM-2. Variable resistance equipment is normally used in the same manner as isotonic equipment.

ISOKINETIC EXERCISE

Isokinetic exercise is dynamic in nature, as are the isotonic and variable resistance methods. The aspect of isokinetic exercise that distinguishes it from the other forms of dynamic exercise is maximum accommodating resistance. The equipment provides resistance equivalent to that which the athlete exerts throughout the entire range of motion for every repetition. This is accomplished by controlling the speed at which the exercise is performed, usually through a hydraulic system. Typically, the athlete exerts a maximum effort on every repetition. The Cybex and Orthotron were the first pieces of equipment to utilize the isokinetic method of exercise.

The advantages of isokinetic exercise over isotonics and variable resistance is speed of exercise. A joint or muscle group can be exercised at slow speeds (30 degrees/second to 60 degrees/second) to stimulate strength gains along the lines of isotonic exercises, or at higher speeds (up to 300 degrees/second) to stimulate strength gains at more functional rates of muscle contraction.

MANUAL RESISTANCE

Often overlooked, manual resistance is a very effective method for strengthening muscles in a rehabilitative setting. It requires no equipment, it is excellent for use in isolating specific muscles, and it can produce isokinetic or near maximum accommodating resistance. Typically, exercise regimens follow a pattern similar to isokinetics, namely, three sets of six to ten repetitions. However, this may vary with the speed of exercise. At faster rates of speed, more repetitions are performed to provide a sufficient work load.

The best method of strengthening muscles following injury is not easily defined. Factors such as postinjury condition, equipment availability, and knowledge and familiarity of the trainer or therapist with various methods all play an important role in determining the best approach. Therefore, the physician must rely on the basic philosophy of increasing strength along with range of motion and allow the methods to be dictated by the patient's needs.

MODALITIES

The total spectrum of physical therapy modalities, from moist heat to ultrasound and high-voltage electrical stimulation, have been used to treat athletic injuries. Each modality, if used appropriately and judiciously, can be a useful adjunct in the rehabilitation process. It must be emphasized that if they are used without regard to the total rehabilitation program or coupled with an aggressive exercise program to recondition the athlete to a highly competitive level, they are of little, if any, value.

Specifically, the use of modalities must be based on several factors:

1. Is the modality safe to use on the injury being treated?

2. Will the modality contribute significantly to the rehabilitation process and the total recovery of the athlete?

3. Is the athletic trainer or therapist trained to use the modality safely and effectively?

The following material is presented in outline form. The specific methods of treatment are not covered in detail. It is recommended that these modalities be used only by properly trained or supervised personnel.

ICE/COLD THERAPY

Ice or cold therapy is the most widely used modality in sports medicine and athletic training. When ice or some other cold substance is placed on an injury a cooling effect takes place. The end result of this cooling effect is a reduction of local blood flow, metabolism, and the reduction of swelling and edema. It also is a very effective local anesthetic.[5]

Indications

Indications for ice or cold therapy include the following: (1) acute and chronic soft tissue injuries such as contusions, strains, and sprains; and (2) relief of pain and muscle spasm.

Contraindications

Contraindications to ice or cold therapy include: (1) cold allergies, circulatory disorders, Raynaud's syndrome, and rheumatoid arthritis; and (2) prolonged use around bony prominences and superficial nerves. Normal treatment time should not exceed 20 minutes, and caution should be used, as frostbite can result from injudicious application of ice.

Methods of Application
Ice.—Crushed ice, ice cubes, or ice flakes can be used. They are usually placed in a plastic bag or commercial rubber/cloth device and held in place or wrapped on with an elastic bandage for 15 to 20 minutes.

Ice Massage.—Large cups of water are frozen and then peeled down to allow the patient or trainer to rub the ice over the injured part, usually for 20 minutes. This is a very economical method of applying ice if a large ice maker is not available.

Chemical and Reusable Cold Packs.—They are handy when ice is not available. However, they are not as effective as cooling agents. They are used the same way as ice packs.

Cold Baths or Whirlpools.—This is a very effective method of cooling large body parts, such as an entire lower leg, or an arm. The temperature should be between 50° and 60° F. Treatment time again is 20 minutes. Caution should be taken not to use water with a temperature below 50° F. "Slush baths" should never be used.

Evaporative Cooling.—Ethyl chloride or fluorimethane sprays are used to cool a superficial area. This is used primarily to relieve pain.

Jobst Cryo/Temp.—This is a device that pumps cold water through an enclosed boot or sleeve that has been applied to an extremity. Temperature and pressure can be controlled. Both constant pressure and intermittent pressure can also be applied. It is very effective in controlling swelling in the acute phase of injury.

HEAT

Heat has been used in a variety of forms to treat athletes since early recorded history. Although the methods have changed with time, the basic effects have not. A local rise in temperature leads to an increased metabolic rate, which in turn leads to more metabolites and heat.[3] As a result of the change in temperature and metabolic production, local blood flow increases to dissipate the heat and to supply additional oxygen to healing tissues. Analgesia, muscle relaxation, and sedation are additional effects of the increase in temperature.

Heat is transferred by several methods:

Conduction.—Heat is conducted from one object to another through the actual contact of the two objects (i.e., hydrocollator pack or heating pad).

Convection.—Convection involves the exchange of heat between a surface and air or fluid moving past the surface (i.e., whirlpool baths).

Radiation.—Heating by radiation involves the transference of energy through space by means of electromagnetic waves (i.e., heat lamps or infrared lamps).

Indications

Local heating is indicated in the treatment of chronic soft tissue injuries. In such cases, local blood flow is needed to reduce edema and increase metabolic production, and local heating will facilitate this. In addition to increasing blood flow, local heating can elevate tissue temperature. Both of these effects are of value, in that they help to increase range of motion and flexibility. Heat aids in the management of local infection and promotes wound healing. Finally, heat is indicated for the relief of muscle spasm, and to produce an analgesic or sedation effect.

Contraindications

Local heating should not be used for acute or subacute injuries, when hemorrhaging or increased swelling is possible; when circulation, sensation, or pain is impaired; or in the case of thermoregulatory disorders.

Methods of Application
Hydrocollator (Moist Heat Packs).—This form of heat therapy is readily available in most training rooms and physical therapy centers. Treatment temperature is recommended between 150° and 165° F. The pack is used over multiple layers of toweling to achieve a comfortable warming effect for 20 minutes.

Whirlpools.—These are usually used for large areas of treatment (i.e., lower leg, total leg, or total arm). Treatment time is the same as for hydrocollator packs. Temperature should never exceed 110° F.

Other forms of heat include shortwave and microwave diathermy, ultrasound, infrared, and paraffin baths. Many are available in training rooms and physical therapy clinics. Indications are similar to those for other heat modalities. However, care must be taken to observe the contraindications as they pertain to each device.

There are a host of other therapeutic modalities that can and are being used to treat athletic injuries. It is our intent to provide a single regimen of rehabilitation for the practitioner. Therefore, we have not emphasized the total spectrum of modalities available to the athletic trainer and physical therapist. We believe that the essential aspect of a rehabilitative program is exercise. The use of modalities to supplement the rehabilitative program is encouraged.

REFERENCES

1. Basmajian JV (ed): *Therapeutic Exercise*, ed 3. Baltimore, Williams & Wilkins Co, 1978, p 127.
2. Hettinger T, Muller EA: Muskelleistung and Muskel training. *Int Angewandte Physiol Arbeitsphysiol* 1953; 15:111–126.
3. Krusen FH (ed): *Handbook of Physical Medicine and Rehabilitation*. Philadelphia, WB Saunders Co, 1966, pp 233–235.
4. Kuprian W (ed): *Physical Therapy for Sports*. Philadelphia, WB Saunders Co, 1981, p 106.
5. Lehman JF (ed): *Therapeutic Heat and Cold*. Baltimore, Williams & Wilkins Co, 1982, pp 563–564.
6. Roy S, Irvin R: *Sports Medicine—Prevention, Evaluation, Management, and Rehabilitation*. Englewood Cliffs, NJ, Prentice-Hall, 1983.
7. Sapega AA, Quedenfeld TC, Moyer RA, et al: Biophysical factors in range of motion exercise. *Phys Sports Med* 1981; 9:57–65.

CHAPTER 2

The Foot

With the advent of the current sports and fitness craze, we have witnessed an increase of injuries to the foot, several of which have been attributed to "overuse." Among these overuse injuries are plantar fasciitis, stress fractures, and retrocalcaneal bursitis.

INJURY: PLANTAR FASCIITIS
Problem: Pain/Inflammation

Plantar fasciitis is characterized by low-grade pain, insidious in onset, located along the medial plantar fascia just distal to the calcaneous.[4] Pain is often felt directly beneath the calcaneous at the insertion of the plantar fascia, and at times on the medial aspect of the calcaneous.[11] It can be experienced while walking and running and, in mild cases, after running. Microtears and inflammation of the plantar fascia are a result of repeated traction of the plantar fascia at its insertion into the calcaneous.[1] This can result from limited ankle dorsiflexion due to a tight gastrocnemius soleus complex.[7] Swelling is not a predominant symptom, yet tenderness is likely to be present.[12]

Ice massage for 20 minutes, several times a day, can help alleviate discomfort temporarily, although it may not be successful for long periods of treatment.[10, 12, 13]

Anti-inflammatory drugs are recommended for the treatment of plantar fasciitis.[1, 10, 12] The injection of steroidal medication at the calcaneal attachment can help control inflammation,[10] but care needs to be taken in cases where symptoms persist in order to avoid local iatrogenic complications.[1] Oral medications can include phenylbutazone (Butazolidin), oxyphenbutazone (Tandearil), indomethacin (Indocin), and ibuprofen (Motrin).[10]

Furey[5] has presented a study of the treatment of 116 patients with plantar fasciitis. The characteristic physical findings were pain and tenderness located in the area of the calcaneal tuberosity. The patients were treated with phenyl-butazone 100 mg four times a day for one week and then three times a day for one week. Heel pads and arch supports were also used. Seventy-one percent of the 78 patients initially treated had excellent or good results after an average follow-up of 5.2 years. Aspirin and other anti-inflammatory agents can be used but none of these agents should be administered without close supervision.[5, 10] Refer to the chapter on medication for a discussion of complications.

The pain that persists in plantar fasciitis can be alleviated with an adhesive strapping known as the low Dye technique. A biomechanical problem, specifically abnormal pronation of the foot, has been identified as possible causal factor for plantar fasciitis.[10, 12] Several authors have recommended the low Dye technique as a means for correcting this problem.[10, 12, 17] Whitesel[17] and Newell[10] state that it stabilizes the head of the first metatarsal by plantar flexing it, and decreases foot pronation. Newell and Miller[10] report that a positive response to this strapping is indicative of mechanical problems and can be used as a guide for prescribing orthotics. The use of moleskin instead of tape is suggested because it is stronger, provides more support, and wears better during exercise.[17]

LOW DYE STRAPPING TECHNIQUE

The low Dye strapping[2] is recommended for treating conditions involving inflammation of the plantar fascia and traumatic or static sprains of the medial and lateral longitudinal arches. It is also recommended for shin splints if the diagnosis is consistent with a musculotendinous inflammation along the medial border of the tibia.

Positioning

The foot is placed in a neutral position with plantar flexion of the first metatarsal ray (Fig 2–1).

Materials

The materials required are 1-in. adhesive tape and 3-in. moleskin. The moleskin is cut to approximate the plantar surface of the foot from just under the metatarsal heads to the calcaneous (Fig 2–2).

Instructions

Step 1.—The moleskin is applied to the metatarsal heads, pulled with slight tension downward through it's midsection, and secured to the calcaneous (Fig 2–3).

Step 2.—Additional support is achieved by applying 1-in. strips of adhesive tape upward from underneath the plantar surface, with equal pressure medially and laterally (Fig 2–4). The length of the tape should not exceed the height of an imaginary line running just beneath the malleoli to the outer borders of the first and fifth metatarsal heads.

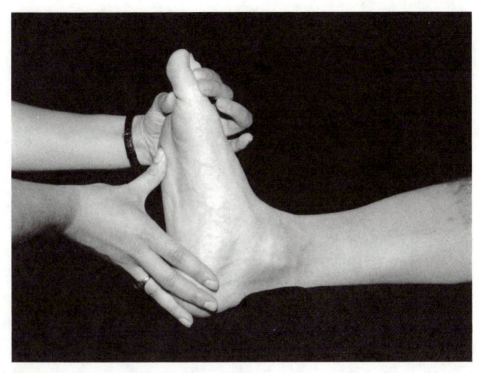

FIG 2–1.
The foot is first placed in a neutral position, with plantar flexion of the first metatarsal ray.

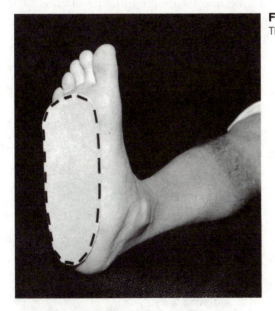

FIG 2–2.
Three-inch moleskin is cut to fit the foot.

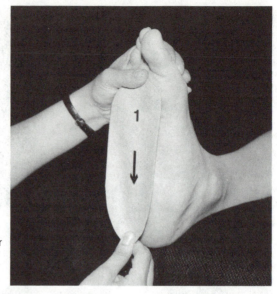

FIG 2–3.
The moleskin is applied to the plantar side of the foot. It extends from just under the metatarsal heads to the calcaneous.

Step 3.—To secure the strapping, the anchor strips are placed over the dorsal aspect of the foot. An additional anchor is placed around the posterior aspect of the calcaneous just beneath the malleoli (Fig 2–5).[2]

ORTHOTIC DEVICES

Orthotic correction is another effective method for treating plantar fasciitis.[10, 12] Similar in function to low Dye strapping, orthotics correct the biomechanical problems responsible for the development of the injury. First, they can correct

FIG 2–4.
The first piece of 1-in. tape is applied. It runs upward underneath the plantar surface, with equal pressure medially and laterally.

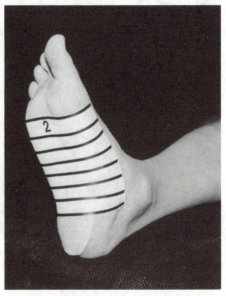

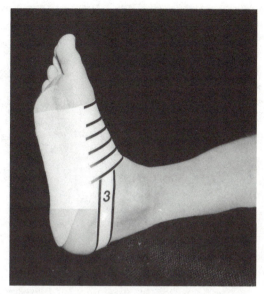

FIG 2–5.
Anchor strips are placed over the dorsal
aspect of the foot to secure the strapping.
An additional anchor is placed around the
posterior aspect of the calcaneous just
beneath the malleoli.

abnormal pronation or pes planus, which stretches the plantar aponeurosis,
leading to fascial strain. Also, in pes cavus, orthotics alleviate the "windlass effect," in which the fascia are tight and there is strain on the calcaneal insertion.
If untreated, the stress on the fascia can lead to the formation of a calcaneal
bone spur. Orthotics serve to maintain the subtalar joint in neutral, and the
midtarsal joint in a stable pronated position[3, 10, 12, 14] (Fig 2–6).

A variety of ready-made arch supports are available in shoe stores and
sporting good stores. However, the erudite and sophisticated runner of today
will usually settle for nothing less than a pair of custom-made orthotic devices,
which cost approximately $275 for prescription and fabrication.

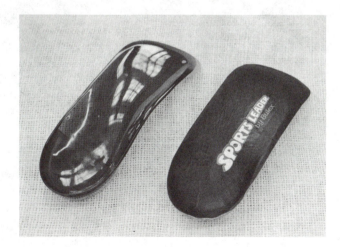

FIG 2–6.
A rigid orthotic, on the left, is used primarily in nonathletic footwear. The sport orthotic *(right)* is more
flexible and used for athletic participation.

The semirigid and rigid runner's orthotic device requires a positive plaster casting or mold of the patient's foot taken with the subtalar joint in a neutral position. Presumably this occurs when the talonavicular joint and forefoot are also in a neutral relationship (Figs 2–7 and 2–8). The plaster positive mold is then sent to the orthotic laboratory for fabrication of the device (Fig 2–9).

The orthosis, in addition to providing rigid support for the medial arch and midfoot, is also "posted" anteriorly and posteriorly in order to support the subtalar joint in a neutral position (Figs 2–10,A and B).[14]

There are some other recommended methods for treating plantar fasciitis. Heel supports, which can either be soft or rigid. Rigid are to be used when pain persists.[1] Arch supports,[4, 7] heel wedges,[4, 7] heel cups, "donuts," and good running shoes[7, 12] are additional methods used to correct biomechanical problems.

REHABILITATION: RANGE OF MOTION/STRETCHING EXERCISES

Several authors advocate stretching exercises for the treatment of plantar fasciitis.[1, 4, 7, 12] Andrews[1] recommends heelcord and plantar fascia exercises. Roy[12] supports stretching of the Achilles tendon. Krissoff and Ferris[7] recommend stretching the gastrocnemius-soleus complex, and the intrinsic and extrinsic musculature of the foot.

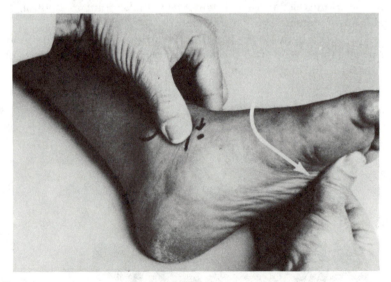

FIG 2–7.
Positive casting for running orthotics should be taken with the subtalar joint in a neutral position. That is, no eversion and no inversion should be present. Presumably, this is determined by ascertaining talonavicular joint congruity by palpating the medial *(arrow)* and dorsolateral aspects of the talonavicular joint with the thumb and forefinger of one hand, then supporting the foot in a neutral position with pressure under the fourth and fifth metatarsal, heads as demonstrated. (From Langer Biomechanics Group, Inc., Deer Park, NY. Used with permission.)

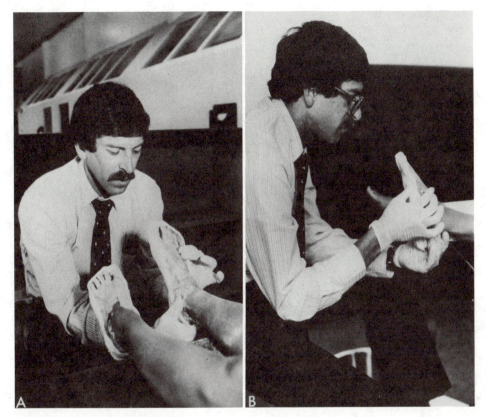

FIG 2–8.
A, casting for runner's orthotics requires palpating the talonavicular joint and maintaining it in a neutral position. **B,** with congruity of the talonavicular joint, the forefoot is maintained in a neutral relationship with the hindfoot by exerting pressure under the fourth and fifth metatarsal heads.

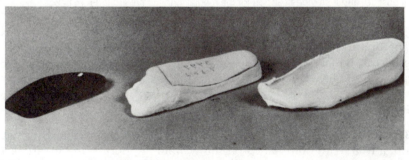

FIG 2–9.
From the positive casting *(right)* a negative impression of the configuration of the plantar surface of the foot is obtained *(center)*. From this, an acrylic rigid orthosis is fabricated *(left)*. (From Langer Biomechanics Group, Inc., Deer Park, NY. Used with permission.)

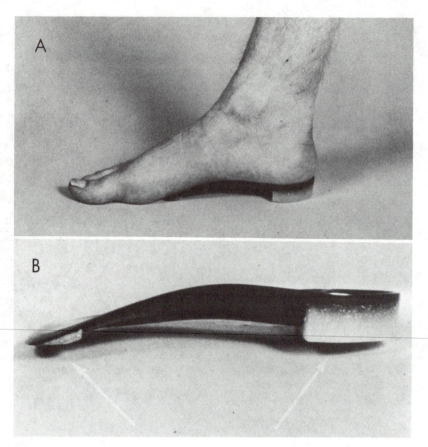

FIG 2–10.
A, viewed from the medial aspect, anterior and posterior heel posts are bonded to the acrylic member. **B,** the runner's orthotic serves two functions: it presumably maintains the subtalar joint in a neutral posture, and it provides support for the medial longitudinal arch. (From Langer Biomechanics Group, Inc., Deer Park, NY. Used with permission.)

The University of Pennsylvania Sports Medicine Center heelcord stretching program can be followed in order to improve ankle range of motion, and gastrocsoleus flexibility. The procedure is as follows:

Heelcord Stretch

1. Stand with feet in a parallel position, toes pointing straight ahead, in front of a wall. With both hands on the wall for support, lean forward, keeping both legs straight. This should create a stretch in the calf (Fig 2–11,A). Hold this for 10 seconds. Return to starting position. Repeat this exercise 15 times, two to three times a day.

2. Repeat the above exercise with bent knees. Stand with feet parallel, bend both knees, and then lean forward (Fig 2–11,B).

3. Repeat both of the above exercises using the heelcord box (Fig 2–11,C and D).

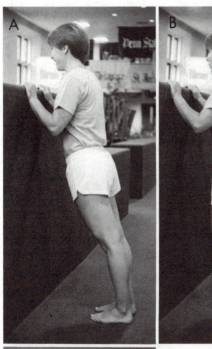

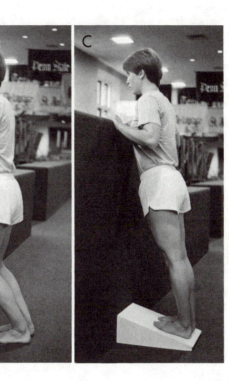

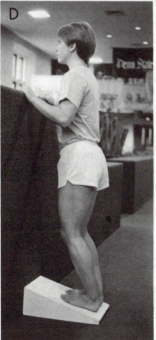

FIG 2–11.
A, the heelcord stretching exercises in the straight leg position can be used to stretch the calf. The stretching position is shown, with the feet parallel and flat on the floor. **B,** heelcord stretch in the bent leg position can be used to improve ankle range of motion. Feet are parallel and remain flat on the floor. **C,** heelcord stretching in the straight leg position using the heelcord box. **D,** heelcord stretching in the bent leg position using the heelcord box.

Rest is often an effective early treatment for overuse injuries. For the treatment of plantar fasciitis, Clancy[4] states that rest is to be continued until there is pain-free palpation, at which point, a gradual training program can be followed. Newell and Miller,[10] and Roy,[12] also prescribe the reduction of activity. Stretching and support are used in combination with rest to provide relief.

Surgical treatment is recommended when conservative management fails. Clancy[4] reported on 15 cases in which the results of surgical release of the plantar fascia were all excellent; the patients returned to running within eight to ten weeks.

INJURY: STRESS FRACTURES
METATARSAL STRESS FRACTURES
Problem: Pain/Disability

Stress fractures are most often observed in individuals who subject their bodies to overtraining, overuse, improper training, or improper equipment. Metatarsal stress fractures can be attributed to a variety of causes. Among them are high force transmitted to the metatarsals during pushoff in the running gate,[7,8] and alterations in shoes, surfaces,[7] training intensity,[7] or foot posture during running. The symptoms that characterize these injuries are ill-defined pain without swelling,[8] focal bony tenderness over the metatarsals, pain along the forepart of the arch, increased pain with weight-bearing and activity, relief of pain through rest, and pain on stretching the plantar arch. Local tenderness and disability are not relieved by the application of pads and heat.[11]

The primary method of treatment is rest. If diagnosed early, metatarsal stress fractures can be treated with relative rest, i.e., discontinuing the activity that caused the injury, thereby avoiding the stress. If the athlete is a runner he or she may maintain conditioning by swimming or bicycling. Return to running should be gradual in order to avoid reinjury.[6,11]

A flexible metatarsal pad or shoe insert can provide effective support for resolving stress fractures.[7] The insert allows the athlete to ambulate normally while providing adequate support for the fracture. The metatarsal pad is constructed of dense foam or plastazote. A firm "insole" is cut for the shoe. A layer of adhesive felt is then positioned on the forefront region and the felt is removed from the area of the affected metatarsal (Fig 2–12). This relief pad removes the weight-bearing from the metatarsal. The pad can be worn as long as necessary for healing to take place, and it can be changed from shoe to shoe.

STRESS FRACTURE OF BASE OF FIFTH METATARSAL

Stress fractures of the base of the fifth metatarsal distal to the tuberosity are classified as: (1) acute fractures, (2) delayed unions, and (3) nonunions.[16]

Torg et al.[15] report that the presence or absence of medullary sclerosis adjacent to the fracture site is an important consideration in deciding the course

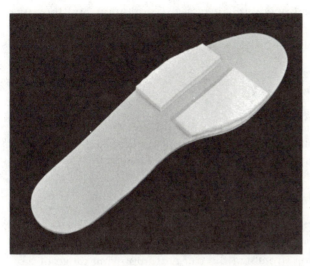

FIG 2–12.
The positioning for an adhesive metatarsal felt pad, used in the treatment of stress fractures, is shown.

of treatment for fractures to the base of the fifth metatarsal distal to the tuberosity. Non–weight-bearing in a plaster boot for six to eight weeks is recommended in acute fractures in which no sclerosis is present. If sclerosis exists, indicating delayed or nonunion, surgery is advocated,[15] followed by non–weight-bearing immobilization.

REHABILITATION: STRETCHING AND STRENGTHENING

Once plaster casting is removed, stretching and strengthening exercises will be required. The specific exercises are described following stress fractures to the tarsal navicular.

STRESS FRACTURES OF THE TARSAL NAVICULAR

Torg et al.[16] reported the results of the treatment of 21 stress fractures of the tarsal navicular.

Symptoms reported by the patients included a history of insidious onset of vague pain in the dorsum of the foot, at the medial aspect of the longitudinal arch, or, in some cases, in both locations. Activity tended to aggravate this ill-defined soreness or cramping sensation. Seventeen of 21 feet had tenderness directly over the tarsal navicular. Swelling, discoloration and limping were not characteristic of this injury.[16] Ten of 21 limbs demonstrated a limited subtalar motion, as well as dorsiflexion.[16]

Torg et al.[16] conclude that the appropriate treatment for acute tarsal navicular stress fracture is immobilization for six to eight weeks in a non–weight-bearing plaster cast. The ten patients in the study who underwent this course of treatment all returned to full activity within three to six months. In contrast, seven out of nine patients who were not placed on a non–weight-bearing regimen were either disabled or experienced repeated fracture.

Those in the study treated operatively because of nonunion, and then immobilized in the non–weight-bearing cast for six to eight weeks returned to full activity in five to seven months.[16]

Problem: Decreased Function

Prolonged immobilization and surgery results in decreased functional ability. Immobilization of the foot and leg results in atrophy, decreased motion, and weakness. Exercises are required to return the ankle and foot to their usual level of functioning.

REHABILITATION: RANGE OF MOTION AND STRETCHING

The heelcord exercises for stretching the calf and improving range of motion are recommended (see Figs 2–11, A-D). For each exercise the stretched position should be held for 10 seconds, and the exercise should be done 15 times, three times a day.

Heelcord Exercises

1. Stand with feet in a parallel position, toes pointing straight ahead, in front of a wall. With both hands on the wall for support, lean forward, keeping both legs straight. There should be a stretch in the calf (see Fig 2–11,A). Hold this for 10 seconds. Return to starting position. Repeat this exercise 15 times, two to three times a day.

2. Repeat the above exercise with bent knees. Stand with feet parallel, bend both knees, and then lean forward (see Fig 2–11,B).

3. Repeat both of the above exercises using the heelcord box (see Fig 2–11,C and D).

REHABILITATION: STRENGTHENING EXERCISES

"Theraband"

"Theraband" exercises for both inversion and eversion should be performed to improve the strength of the musculature in the lower leg. Ten to 15 repetitions of each exercise should be done, once a day. The detailed description and corresponding illustrations can be found in Chapter 3 (see Figs 3–24 and 3–25).

Eversion (Outward).—With the "Theraband" attached around both feet, and with the feet dorsiflexed (up), move feet apart, and return. Repeat, 10 to 15 times. With feet in neutral position (90 degrees), move feet apart, and return. Repeat, 10 to 15 times (see Figs 3–24,A and B).

Inversion (Inward).—With feet crossed, and the "Theraband" attached around them, move feet apart, and return. Repeat, 10 to 15 times (see Figs 3–25,A and B).

Heel and Toe Walking

1. Stand on toes and walk as long as possible, up to five minutes. Repeat two times per day.

2. Walk on heels for as long as possible, up to five minutes. Repeat two times per day.

3. If soreness develop, use ice for about 20 minutes following each of these exercise sessions.

REHABILITATION: PROPRIOCEPTION AND AGILITY EXERCISES

Even after the patient has regained motion and function they will still have proprioceptive and agility deficits. Proprioception can be improved with wobbleboard exercises and agility through an agility program similar to the one outlined in Chapter 3.

Wobbleboard Exercises

Exercises should be performed for plantar flexion, dorsiflexion, inversion, eversion, pronation, and supination on the unidirectional wobbleboard, and through the range of motion on the multidirectional wobbleboard. Exercises should be done once a day, seven days a week. Refer to the illustrations of these exercises (see Figs 3–39 and 3–40).

Exercises on the Unidirectional Wobbleboard.—For each of the exercises described below, the athlete is instructed to rock back and forth in a controlled manner, three minutes in each direction. When exercising the injured leg, the patient is to stand on that leg only. A wall or a chair should be used for support.

Exercises for Plantar and Dorsiflexion.—Follow the steps below.

1. Place the injured foot on the wobbleboard with the axis running perpendicular to the foot (see Fig 3–39,A).
2. Rock back and forth, touching the front edge to the floor, then the back edge, and so on.

Exercises for Inversion and Eversion.—Follow the steps below.

1. Place the injured foot on the wobbleboard with the axis running vertical to the foot (see Fig 3–39,B).
2. Rock back and forth in a controlled manner, touching the right edge to the floor, and then left edge, and so on.

Exercises for Supination and Pronation in 45 Degrees External Rotation.—Follow the steps below.

1. Place the foot on the wobbleboard diagonally, as shown in Figure 3–39,C.
2. Rock back and forth, touching first the right edge to the floor and then the left edge and so on.

Exercises for Supination and Pronation at 45 Degrees Internal Rotation.—Follow the steps below.

1. Place the foot on the wobbleboard diagonally as shown in Figure 3–39,D.
2. See step 2 above.

Exercises Using the Multidirectional Wobbleboard.—Follow the steps below.

1. Place the injured leg on the multidirectional board.
2. Using a wall or chair for support, rotate the ankle clockwise, rolling the edge close to, but not touching the floor.
3. Repeat step 2, rotating the ankle in the opposite direction (see Figs 3–40,A and B).

Agility Exercises

The following are agility exercises that can be performed (refer to Chapter 3 for the detailed outline and illustrations): rope skipping, straight ahead jogging, straight ahead running, backward running, running circles (5 yd in diameter): clockwise and counterclockwise, 90 degree cuts while running, running zigzags at 45 degrees, and other sports-specific agility and skill activities.

INJURY: RETROCALCANEAL BURSITIS
Problem: Pain/Inflammation

Retrocalcaneal bursitis is due to an inflammation of the bursal tissues that surround the insertion of the Achilles tendon at the calcaneous.[7, 1] Retrocalcaneal bursitis can be due to the irritation from a poorly fitted or flimsy heel counter in an athletic shoe.[1, 7] In addition to external pressure, either overuse or irritation of the bony prominence can contribute to the development of bursitis.[4] Pain is a prominent symptom,[9] and is experienced either at the superior aspect of the calcaneous,[4] or anterior to the insertion of the Achilles tendon between the posterior malleolus and the tendon.[13] Swelling may also occur.[4]

Cryotherapy can be used to treat this injury (see Chapters 1, 3, and 12).

Retrocalcaneal bursitis can be treated with a steroid injection into the bursal tissue.[4, 7, 13] Injections should be made behind the tendon,[4] not into it, as this can interfere with the regenerative process, and predispose the tendon to injury by weakening it.[9] Kulund supports this, explaining that steroids can suppress collagen synthesis.[8] Chronic symptoms may be temporarily treated with

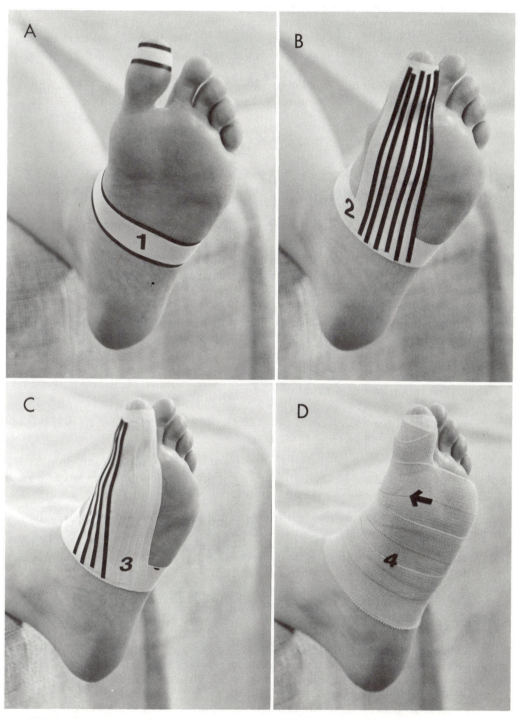

FIG 2–13.
Adhesive strapping for turf toe. **A,** the anchor strips are applied. **B,** the strips to maintain the foot in neutral are applied to the plantar surface of the foot. **C,** additional strips on the medial side are applied. **D,** an adhesive bandage is then used to enclose the tape application.

medication. Oral anti-inflammatory medications can be used,[13] and discussion of their use and that of steroidal medications can be found in Chapter 12.

The use of heel lifts can also be effective.[1, 7, 9, 13] The heel lift acts to remove the stretch on the tendon and elevates the heel to help relieve the irritation from the shoe.

Shields[13] recommends rest for two weeks. If the combination of rest with other modes of conservative treatment does not prove successful then surgery may be necessary.

INJURY: TURF TOE
Problem: Pain/Swelling

Turf toe refers to a sprain of the metatarsal phalangeal joint of the great toe. Pain occurs in the injured plantar joint capsule when the toe is hyperextended.[8] Ice, again, is an effective therapeutic agent for the relief of acute pain associated with turf toe. Withdrawal from the activity that elicited the injury will provide relief and enable healing to occur. Turf toe can be treated with adhesive strapping, and/or firmer shoes with a spring steel or Orthoplast forefoot splint to reduce forefoot motion and extension of the great toe (Fig 2–13,A–D).

TURF TOE STRAPPING

The taping procedure is as follows:

1. Anchor strips are placed around the great toe and another around the midsection of the foot (see Fig 2–13,A).

2. Six strips should be placed on the plantar surface of the foot, running from the anchor at the big toe to the anchor at the midsection. These strips are to maintain the big toe in the neutral position (see Fig 2–13,B).

3. Several more strips can run from the big toe to the midsection on the medial side (see Fig 2–13,C).

4. Adhesive Ace bandage is then wrapped around the big toe and the foot in the clockwise direction, as shown in Fig 2–13,D.

REFERENCES

1. Andrews JR: Overuse syndromes of the lower extremity. *Clin Sports Med* 1983; 2:137.
2. Bonci CM: Adhesive strapping techniques. *Clin Sports Med* 1982; 1:99–116.
3. Campbell JW, Inman VT: Treatment of plantar fasciitis and calcaneal spurs with the UC-BL shoe insert. *Clin Orthop* 1974; 103:57–62.
4. Clancy WG: Runner's injuries: II. Evaluation and treatment of specific injuries. *Am J Sports Med* 1980; 8(4):287–289.
5. Furey JG: Plantar fasciitis: The painful heel syndrome. *J Bone Joint Surg Am* 1975; 57:672–673.

6. Gregg JK, Das M: Foot and ankle problems in preadolescent and adolescent athletes. *Clin Sports Med* 1982; 1:131–147.
7. Krissoff WB, Ferris WD: Runner's injuries. *Phys Sports Med* 1979; 7(12):53–64.
8. Kulund DN: The leg, ankle, and foot, in Kulund DN (ed): *The Injured Athlete.* Philadelphia, JB Lippincott Co, 1982 pp 425–472.
9. Leach RE, James S, Wasilewski S: Achilles tendonitis. *Am J Sports Med* 1981; 9(2):93–98.
10. Newell SG, Miller SJ: Conservative treatment of plantar fascial strain. *Phys Sports Med* 1977; 9(2):68–73.
11. O'Donaghue DH: Injuries of the foot, in O'Donaghue DH (ed): *Treatment of Injuries to Athletes.* Philadelphia, WB Saunders Co, 1984, pp 641–668.
12. Roy S: How I manage plantar fasciitis. *Phys Sports Med* 1983; 11:127–131.
13. Shields CL: Achilles tendon injuries and disabling conditions. *Phys Sports Med* 1982; 10(12):77–84.
14. Torg JS: Athletic footwear and orthotic appliances. *Clin Sports Med* 1982; 1:157–175.
15. Torg JS, Balduini FC, Zelko RR, et al: Fractures of the base of the fifth metatarsal distal to the tuberosity. *J Bone Joint Surg Am* 1984; 66:209–214.
16. Torg JS, Pavlov H, Cooley LH, et al: Stress fractures of the tarsal navicular. *J Bone Joint Surg Am* 1982; 64:700–712.
17. Whitesel J, Newell SG: Modified low Dye strapping. *Phys Sports Med* 1980; 8(9):129–130.

CHAPTER 3

The Ankle

The ankle is one of the most frequently injured joints in athletes.[15, 25] Most of these injuries are nonsurgical cases; thus, the need for rehabilitation procedures targeted at the many problems that can arise is evident. Approximately 10% to 30% of all injuries are ankle injuries.[25] According to Dameron,[5] estimations indicate that out of a group of 10,000 persons, approximately 365 sprains will occur per year, depending on the amount of participation in athletic activities. Five percent to 10% of the injuries seen at the University of Pennsylvania Sports Medicine Center are ankle sprains.[25] This chapter defines (1) the different problems accompanying injuries to the ankle, (2) the goals toward which treatment is aimed, and (3) the corresponding, step-by-step treatment procedure.

Problem: Pain

Pain occurs with all degrees of ankle injuries. Three recommended treatment procedures administered to alleviate it are immobilization, ice, and medication.

Immobilization as a method of treatment for ligamentous injuries to the ankle and foot has been a matter of debate.[3, 8–10, 15, 17] While immobilization formerly constituted the treatment protocol following surgery and severe injuries, studies have been conducted that illustrate that immobilization may not necessarily be beneficial or significantly further recovery.[8–10, 15] A consensus has developed among some physicians that mobilization is the treatment of choice [8–10] for severe as well as mild injuries. We recommend immobilization for the treatment of the pain that accompanies moderate and severe ankle injuries. In addition to alleviating pain by restricting movement, immobilization also reduces edema and associated swelling. There are three forms of immobilization: adhesive strapping, air splints, and plaster casting.

Jackson et al.,[15] in the study of 105 ankle injuries sustained by cadets at U.S. Military Academy, observed that the functional recovery period for those treated

with plaster immobilization was longer than for those not immobilized. An unpublished pilot study performed in 1972 indicated that the amount of time recovery was prolonged corresponded approximately to the number of days the ankle remained immobilized.[15]

The work of Brostrom[3] has been cited as most significant.[24] He compared 95 cases of surgical repair and plaster immobilization, 82 cases of immobilization without surgery, and 104 cases of adhesive strapping and early mobilization. Surgical repair showed the best results. Only 3 of 95 surgically treated patients reported symptoms of ankle instability, and the anterior drawer sign was observed in only 5% of these cases, while 20% of the nonsurgically treated groups demonstrated instability, and 30% of them were found to have the anterior drawer sign. The report concluded that there were no verifiable differences observed between the plaster immobilization group and the strapping group. Surgical treatment was not recommended routinely in the treatment of ankle sprains because of the overload that it would place on surgical units, and to the risk of surgical complications with osteoarthritis. While there were no long-term differences between the plaster group and the strapping group, plaster immobilization led to longer absence from work. Brostrom recommends strapping as the more favorable of the two treatments. In the case of plaster immobilization, he recommends a one- or two-week period, stating that longer immobilization periods did not seem to improve progress.

ADHESIVE STRAPPING

The need for support or immobilization is dependent on the individual's ability to bear weight. In cases of mild disability the individual is best supported by an open Gibney adhesive strapping, in the acute stage, followed by a modified Gibney adhesive strapping after swelling begins to subside. The application procedures for both of these techniques are described below.[1] The general principles for taping can be found in the section on instability, and should be reviewed.

Open Gibney Technique

This adhesive strapping (Fig 3–1) is used therapeutically after acute ankle injuries to help control swelling and lend support to the ankle joint. The strapping is characterized by a 1-in. wide incomplete tape enclosure along the anterior portion of the foot and lower leg. This allows for expansion of the joint if increased swelling develops and decreases the possibility of circulatory impairment and soft tissue constriction. The strapping outlined is indicated for injuries to the lateral ligamentous structures.

Positioning.—The foot is placed in a neutral position with slight eversion (Fig 3–2,A).

Materials.—The materials required are 1½-in. adhesive tape and a ¼-in. adhesive felt or foam horseshoe. The horseshoe is cut to approximate the contours of the lateral malleolus and is applied accordingly (Fig 3–2,B).

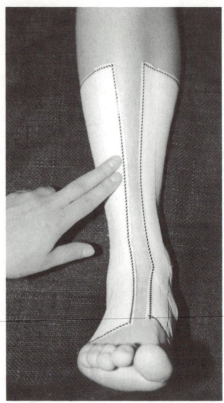

FIG 3–1.
The open Gibney strapping technique is shown.

Step 1.—Application of the tape begins with an anchor strip placed just beneath the musculotendinous junction of the calf. The contour of this portion of the lower leg dictates angling of the tape upward to prevent gapping. A second anchor strip is applied by encircling the arch just proximal to the metatarsal heads (Fig 3–3,A).

Step 2.—A stirrup is then applied in a medial to lateral direction, beginning and ending at the calf anchor. The tape is directed behind the malleoli and runs parallel to the Achilles tendon (Fig 3–3,B).

Step 3.—A Gibney strip is then placed horizontally around the periphery of the foot just beneath the malleoli. The tape is pulled medially to laterally, beginning and ending at the foot anchor (Fig 3–3,C).

Step 4.—Repeat application of at least two more stirrups and accompanying Gibney strips as indicated in steps 1 and 2, by overlapping the tape by a half width. A basketweave pattern will result (Fig 3–3,D).

Step 5.—The strapping is completed by continuing the Gibney strips up the lower leg to the calf-anchor. Two or three incomplete circular strips are also

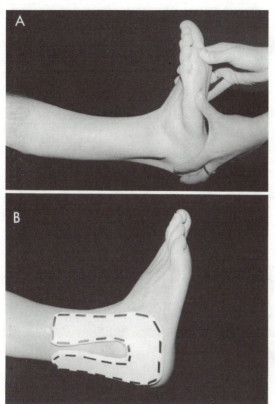

FIG 3–2.
A, for the open Gibney strapping technique the foot is placed in a neutral position with slight eversion. **B,** an adhesive felt or foam horseshoe is applied first.

applied around the arch (Fig 3–3,E). After completion of the strapping, an elastic bandage can be applied from the base of the toes to the calf for added compression.

Closed Gibney Technique

This taping technique, pictured in Figure 3–4, helps to decrease the risk of potential reinjury to the ankle joint following an inversion or eversion sprain. It is also recommended for those athletes who present with complaints of chronic ankle instability. The strapping presented is indicated for an inversion, plantar-flexion injury.

Positioning.—Positioning is the same as for the open Gibney technique (see Fig 3–2,A).

Materials.—The materials required are a pretaping underwrap, lubricated gauze pads, and 1½-in. adhesive tape.

Step 1.—The skin, which has been shaved, is prepared with lubricated gauze pads and underwrap (Fig 3–5).

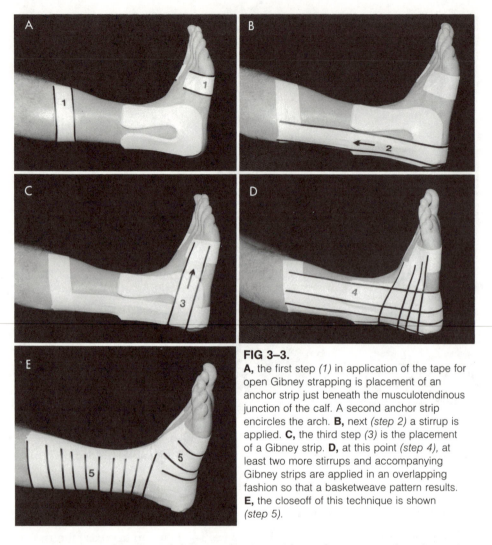

FIG 3–3.
A, the first step *(1)* in application of the tape for open Gibney strapping is placement of an anchor strip just beneath the musculotendinous junction of the calf. A second anchor strip encircles the arch. **B,** next *(step 2)* a stirrup is applied. **C,** the third step *(3)* is the placement of a Gibney strip. **D,** at this point *(step 4)*, at least two more stirrups and accompanying Gibney strips are applied in an overlapping fashion so that a basketweave pattern results. **E,** the closeoff of this technique is shown *(step 5)*.

Step 2.—Application of the tape begins with anchor strips placed just beneath the musculotendinous junction of the gastrocnemius-soleus group. Each strip is angled upward and overlaps the preceding one by a half width (Fig 3–6,A).

Step 3.—Stirrups are then applied in a medial to lateral direction, beginning and ending at the calf anchor. The first stirrup is directed behind the malleoli and runs parallel to the Achilles tendon. Each consecutive strip is worked toward the toes and overlaps the previous one by a half width (Fig 3–6,B).

Step 4.—The stirrups are reanchored (Fig 3–6,C).

Step 5.—The figure-of-eight anchor begins medially at the malleolus (Fig 3–7,A). The tape is pulled under the arch and up and around the outside of the

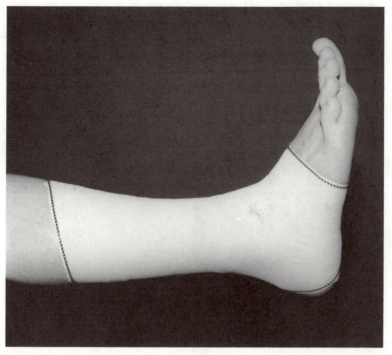

FIG 3–4.
The closed Gibney strapping technique is shown.

foot, staying just behind the base of the fifth metatarsal (Fig 3–7,B). The upper portion of the figure-of-eight is completed by directing the tape horizontally around the distal aspect of the tibia and fibula (Fig 3–7,C). The tape will crisscross the lower portion of the eight anteriorly at the ankle joint and end at the medial malleolus.

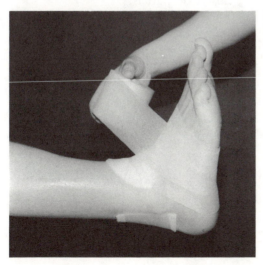

FIG 3–5.
The skin is first shaved and then prepared with lubricated gauze pads and under wrap *(step 1)*.

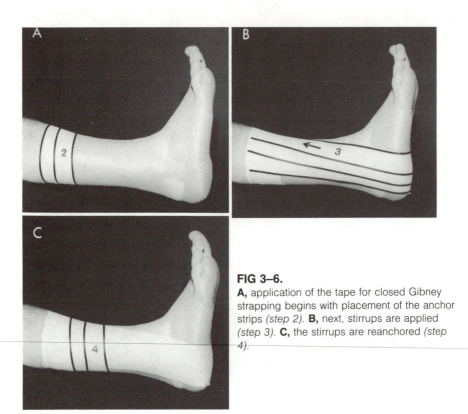

FIG 3–6.
A, application of the tape for closed Gibney strapping begins with placement of the anchor strips *(step 2).* **B,** next, stirrups are applied *(step 3).* **C,** the stirrups are reanchored *(step 4).*

Step 6.—A lateral heel lock begins medially at the calf anchors, passes diagonally downward behind the lateral malleolus, and crosses the Achilles tendon (Fig 3–8,A). The tape then passes down the inside of the calcaneous (Fig 3–8,B), under and around the outside of the foot (Fig 3–8,C), and ends at the medial aspect of the calf anchors. A medial heel lock is applied in the same manner with a reversal of the previously described pattern.

Step 7.—The close-off procedure begins with three to four horizontal strips placed around the periphery of the foot. The first strip is applied beneath the malleoli and each consecutive strip overlaps the previous one by a half width. The procedure continues by circumferential application of tape up the lower leg to the calf anchor (Fig 3–9,A).

Step 8.—Two to three close-off strips are also circled around the arch (Fig 3–9,B).

Step 9.—The strapping is completed by application of a figure-of-eight strip as outlined in step 3 (Fig 3–9,C).

Step 10.—The tape is removed by cutting along the medial aspect of the foot, behind the malleolus, and up along the medial aspect of the tibia (Fig 3–10).

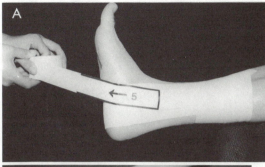

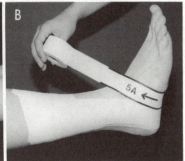

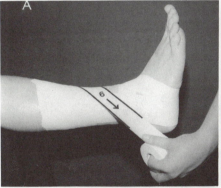

FIG 3–7.
Step 5 in the closed Gibney technique consists of wrapping the tape in a figure-of-eight pattern. **A,** the figure-of-eight begins medially at the malleolus. **B,** for the lower half of the figure-of-eight, the tape is pulled under the arch and up and around the outside of the foot *(step 5A)*. **C,** the upper portion of the figure-of-eight is formed by wrapping the tape around the distal aspect of the tibia and fibula *(step 5B)*.

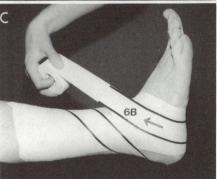

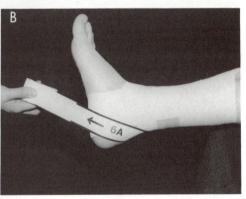

FIG 3–8.
Step 6 in the closed Gibney technique. **A,** lateral heel lock begins medially at calf anchors, passes diagonally downward behind the lateral malleolus, and crosses the Achilles tendon. **B,** tape then is passed down the inside of the calcaneus *(step 6A)*. **C,** tape is passed under and around the outside of the foot and ends at the medial aspect of the calf anchors *(step 6B)*.

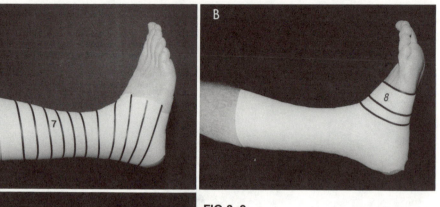

FIG 3–9.
The close-off procedure for the closed Gibney technique. **A,** three to four horizontal strips are placed around the periphery of the foot, beginning just beneath the malleoli. Consecutive strips are applied, each one overlapping the previous one by a half width, and circumferential application of tape continues up the lower leg to the calf anchor *(step 7).* **B,** two to three close-off strips are circled around the arch *(step 8).* **C,** strapping is completed by the application of figure-of-eight strip *(step 9).*

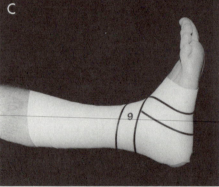

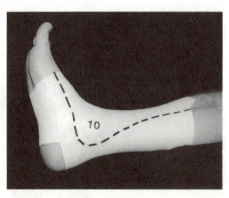

FIG 3–10.
The cutting pattern for removing tape is shown *(step 10).* Tape is removed by cutting along the medial aspect of the foot, behind the malleolus, and up along the medial aspect of the tibia.

Air-Stirrup

A second medium for immobilizing the ankle is the Air-Stirrup.

Stover[24] developed the Air-Stirrup as an alternative to adhesive strapping (Fig 3–11). It consists of two segments of Orthoplast about 3 to 4 in. wide, which run along the lateral and medial sides of the ankle, and are connected by a padded heel piece. The outer shells contain inner-lining air bags, which are inflatable via plastic tubing and are self-sealable. The stirrup can be worn comfortably with an athletic shoe. The value of the Air-Stirrup is its ability to provide protection by limiting inversion (Fig 3–12) while simultaneously allowing dorsi

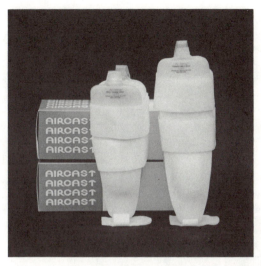

FIG 3–11.
Aircast standard ankle brace *(right)*.
Aircast ankle training brace *(left)*.

and plantar flexion (Fig 3–13). It can be used to treat lateral ligamentous injuries, as well as a host of other injuries that require lateral and medial support. The splint can be used either as a primary treatment for sprains and fractures or as a secondary treatment following earlier plaster removal.

The following are the instructions for the initial application of the Air-Stirrup, as recommended by the manufacturer.

The Air-Stirrup Ankle Training Brace initially requires a few customizing adjustments. Reapplication requires only tightening of the straps. The air cells are preinflated and normally will not require further attention. However, a tube is furnished for inflation by mouth, if necessary. An absorbent sock should be worn for comfort, and a laced shoe for maximum support.

1. Adjust the heel width. The two sides are connected at the heel with Velcro. Adjust the width so the sides are snug but not tight. Peel back the tip of the air cells for access. Keep heel pad centered (Fig 3–14,A).

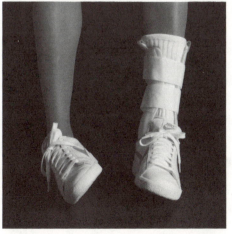

FIG 3–12.
The Aircast ankle training brace, worn with a tennis shoe, limits inversion.

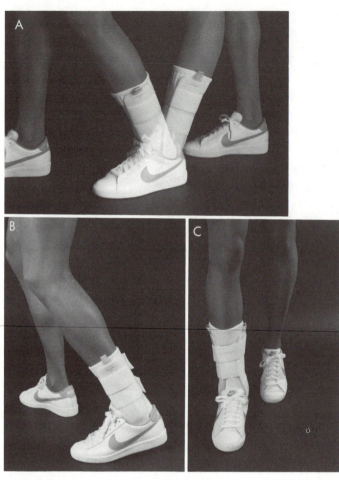

FIG 3–13.
A-C, Aircast ankle training brace permits dorsiflexion.

2. Wrap bottom strap distally. Put on and lace up shoe (Fig 3–14,B).

3. Wrap top strap around, spiraling upward to lie flat. Be certain the side panels are centered along the leg and ankle (Fig 3–14,C).

4. Pressurize the preinflated air cells. Squeeze the sides together with one hand while tightening each strap. Tighten until comfortable but avoid excessive compression (Fig 3–14,D).

5. For removal, release the straps only on the medial side. This will preserve the initial adjustment (Fig 3–14,E).

For reapplication, slip on the preadjusted brace and repeat the pressurization of step 3.

After a half hour or so the brace may feel loose from the displacement of excess fluid from the leg. Retighten until comfortable.

If there is pinching or the presence of a pressure point, loosen the straps

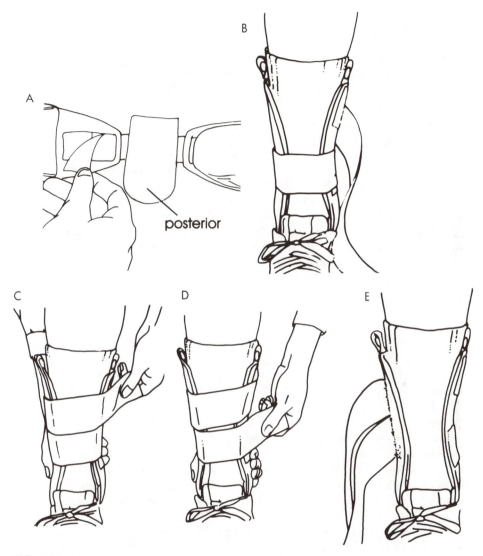

FIG 3–14.
A, adjust the heel width. **B,** adjust the wraparound straps. **C,** spiral straps to conform to ankle. **D,** pressurize the preinflated air cells. **D,** to remove, release the straps on the medial side.

and repeat step 2, repositioning the sides. If the pressure point persists, add a small amount of air to that side. Insert the filling tube about 1½ in. into the valve. Blow with steady pressure. Seal by squeezing the valve flat just below the tube end while slowly withdrawing the tube. Fold and close the valve.

   Maintenance.—The brace can be hand-washed in lukewarm water with a mild soap or detergent. Air dry with artificial heat. If a heel pad should become worn, or an air cell punctured (this occurs in fewer than 1%), please call Aircast (toll free) for prompt replacement.

Note.—At high altitudes the lower atmospheric pressure will expand the air cells beyond their optimal ¼ in. level. Adjust by inserting the filling tube and squeezing out the excess air. With the valve open, the foam liner will expand to the proper level. Then reseal the valve.

When flying, simply readjust the strap to a comfortable pressure.

The Ankle Training Brace is manufactured by Aircast Inc. (P.O. Box T, Summit, NJ 07901), and purchase includes a warranty policy.

PLASTER CASTING

In individuals who require slightly more rigid support, an Unna boot made of Dome-Paste bandage (Dome Laboratories, West Haven, Conn.) is warranted.

Rigid casting is reserved for those individuals who are unable to bear weight following a grade 2 or grade 3 injury. Typically, a short-leg weight-bearing cast is applied for one to three weeks. During cast immobilization, strength in the upper leg and hip of the limb will decrease. Therefore, an exercise program designed to maintain strength must be instituted.

CRYOTHERAPY

It is important to remember that cold therapy can and should be continued while the ankle is immobilized. Cold will penetrate tape, Dome-Paste, and plaster or fiberglass casts.

Cryotherapy, or the use of cold, is the second modality to be implemented in treating the pain associated with ankle injuries. Its action as a local anesthetic is discussed in Chapter 12.

Hocutt et al.[14] compared the use of cryotherapy to heat therapy in the treatment of 37 ankle sprains of varying severity. Cryotherapy consisted of ice whirlpool (40° to 50° F) for 12 to 20 minutes, one to three times a day, or the use of an ice pack for 15 to 20 minutes, one to three times a day. Heat therapy consisted of soaking the ankle in a warm bath, or applying a heat pack for approximately 15 minutes, one to three times a day. They concluded that those treated with cryotherapy early, within 36 hours, returned to full activity on an average of about 15 days earlier than those treated with cryotherapy late, after 36 hours, usually up to 48 hours, or heat therapy, either early or late. It took 13.2 days for those with grade 4 sprains to return to activity if treated with cryotherapy early. If cryotherapy was not begun until after 36 hours, the recovery period extended to 30.4 days. Comparisons were made between patients with grade 3 sprains who were treated with cryotherapy early, cryotherapy late, and heat therapy early. If cryotherapy was begun within 36 hours of injury, patients were able to run and jump without pain in six days. If cryotherapy did not begin until after 36 hours of injury, pain-free running and jumping were not possible for 11 days. Those treated with heat therapy early took 14.8 days to return to running and jumping.

The use of cold in the acute and follow-up stages of the athletic injury is well-documented by Kalenak,[16] McMaster,[20] and Vegso and Harmon.[25] A detailed description of the physiological effects of cold are presented in Chapter 12. Initial treatment consists of application of ice, compression, and elevation.

The procedure for application of cold is as follows:

1. Apply the ice to the affected area as soon as possible after rehabilitative exercise.

2. Apply the ice for 20 to 25 minutes. This is the maximum time for one ice application.

3. If the ice is to be repeated after the initial application, a 45-minute rest period is needed.

4. Cold is best applied to the ankle by using an icebag, cold whirlpool, or Jobst Cryo/Temp system (Fig 3–16).

5. When using ice or a cold whirlpool, the whole joint or muscular area should be covered.

6. In the acute stage, elevate the area above the heart during the cold application procedure when possible.

7. Due to ice application, the patient may feel the following sensations on the affected area: cold, burning, pain, and numbness. These sensations decrease in magnitude as the body becomes accustomed to cold.

After the ice is taken off, the area will be red; it will return to normal color in 15 to 20 minutes.

Medication is yet another way in which pain can be treated. Aspirin and phenylbutazone (Butazolidin) are pharmacological agents commonly used in the treatment of acute ankle injuries. Indication, dosage, rationale for treatment, and contraindications are discussed in Chapter 12.

Problem: Swelling

Swelling is associated with most levels of ankle injuries (Fig 3–15). It can, however, be differentiated into two types: acute and chronic. The treatment procedure varies somewhat for each form of swelling.

Acute Swelling

The appropriate initial treatment regimen consists of application of ice, compression, and elevation. This is easily recalled by the mnemonic "ICE," as mentioned by Brown.[4]

Physiologically, cold causes vasoconstriction, thereby decreasing local blood flow and hemorrhage, with resultant decrease of edema. Additionally, cold acts as a local anesthetic, which aids in the control of pain and secondarily to relieve muscle spasm. Heat is an absolute contraindication for acute swelling. Unfortunately, it is still routinely prescribed after 24 hours. Heat is a vasodilator. It increases the amount of swelling, which contributes to a longer period of healing.

We recommend that heat should never be used in the acute or subacute phases of recovery.

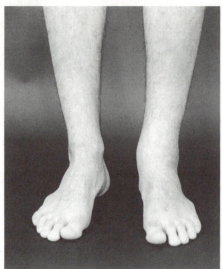

FIG 3–15.
An anterior view of a grade II lateral ankle sprain
demonstrates swelling.

Jobst Cryo/Temp System

The Jobst Cryo/Temp cold and pressure therapy system is recommended
in the treatment of acute swelling. This device allows for the application of cold
with intermittent or constant pressure. This is accomplished via a flow of coolant to an appliance that encloses the extremity (Fig 3–16). There are a variety of
appliances available for use on all extremity injuries.

The temperature can be adjusted to range from room temperature to 34° F.
The pressure can be set between 0 and 160 mm Hg, and can be applied constantly or intermittently, from 0 to 180 seconds on, 0 to 60 seconds off.*

Starkey[22] supports the use of cold (37° F), or cryotherapy, for the initial stage
of treatment. His study explored the use of a modality that combined cold treatment, exercise, and massage, and was designed to assist in venous return. A
massage unit that provides compression, cold, massage through alternating
pressure, and allows for dorsal and plantar flexion, and full range of motion,
was applied to 13 ankles that had suffered inversion sprains. The time period
for one cycle of pressure application and pressure release was 15 seconds, and
the average overall treatment time was 30 minutes. He concludes that recovery
time was decreased by two days as compared to the normal ice, compression,
and elevation treatment, and that this was due only to the fact that cold, massage, and elevation were combined.

Application of the Jobst Cryo/Temp System.—The application procedure
for the Jobst is as follows:

1. The injured leg should be placed into the appliance. Leg appliances
range from half-leg to three-quarter-leg and full-leg appliances. The three-
quarter-leg appliance is shown here (see Fig 3–16).

*Jobst Institute instructional literature.

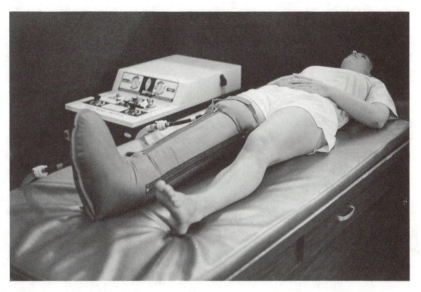

FIG 3–16.
The application of the Jobst three-quarter leg appliance is shown.

2. The treatment temperature is normally set between 55° and 70° F.

3. The recommended treatment pressure is set between 80 and 120 mm Hg and applied for 20 minutes.

4. The treatment is continued for 20 minutes. The pressure is run intermittently with an on time-off time ratio of 3:1.

5. Jobst treatments may be repeated several times per day.

Chronic Swelling

The following are treatment modes for chronic swelling: moist heat packs, warm whirlpool baths, contrast baths, compression stockings, electrogalvanic stimulation (EGS), artherocentesis (joint aspiration), and intraarticular steroid injections.

While acute swelling is to be treated with ice, heat can be used for chronic swelling. Moist heat packs, warm whirlpools, and contrast baths are all forms of heat therapy that work via conduction. In a simplified form, the mechanism for thermotherapy is as follows: the increase in temperature leads to an increase in metabolism. The resulting increase of metabolic products leads to dilation of the arterioles, which allows for an increase in blood flow bringing nutrients and protective elements.[13, 22] This is thought to have a beneficial effect.[4] In addition to increasing local circulation, heat is also indicated to relieve pain, due to its analgesic effect, and to prepare the injured area for exercise.[23]

McCluskey et al.[19] recommend heat therapy once active swelling has been controlled and range of motion has increased. Their protocol consists of contrasts baths, alternating between four minutes of warm whirlpool (100° to 104° F) and one minute of ice bath (47° F).[19]

Hydrocolator packs and warm whirlpool baths may be applied for 20 minutes at temperatures of 100° to 106° F, two to three times a day.[19, 21]

Electrogalvanic stimulation is a modality widely employed to reduce swelling. It acts as an electrical and mechanical aid in stimulating venous and lymphatic return.

Aspiration and Injection

Frequently, ankle sprains develop effusions that require aspiration, often yielding up to 5 ml of synovial fluid or blood. In addition to the aspiration, a single injection of corticosteroid such as triamcinolone acetonide suspension (Kenalog-10) into the joint has been found to be extremely effective in controlling the inflammatory response and reducing chronic swelling.[25]

In an attempt to document the possibility that aspiration injection treatment lessens morbidity and reduces the period of incapacitation, Brady and Arnold[2] compared the effects of two different treatment procedures on 47 ankle sprains with talar tilts of 6 degrees or less. The control group of 11 patients received conservative treatment consisting of application of ice compresses for 48 to 72 hours, adhesive strapping for five days, supportive shoes, and early ambulation. The experimental group of 36 patients received 48 to 72 hours of ice pack therapy, followed by aspiration of blood, over the medial and lateral cornices, and the injection of the periarticular structures with hyaluronidase-lidocaine solution. Recovery was defined as the time at which the injured ankle regained motion equivalent to that of the uninjured ankle, when swelling was no longer present, and when the patient could run and jump without pain. The recovery time for the members of the control group was as follows: the average time was six weeks, the shortest being three weeks and the longest being nine weeks. One case of reinjury occurred in the control group. In the experimental group, 7 of 37 returned to football in one week, 27 returned in two weeks. Two patients were immobilized following the injection treatment and they returned after three weeks. Twelve patients in the experimental group required a second aspiration. Reinjury results for the experimental group were as follows: two suffered reinjury following return to activity; one athlete was reinjured four months after treatment, three within the same season, following treatment, and one a year later.

Zoltan[26] compared a control group of 54 patients to an experimental group of 45 patients for the difference in recovery time from ankle sprains. The control group was treated with ice, compression, elevation, and early immobilization. The experimental group received the same, but in addition their ankles were aspirated and injected with 4 to 10 ml of 1% lidocaine. The experimental group underwent aspiration in the manner described by Brady and Arnold. The end point for recovery was set as the time when the patient could return to normal everyday activities. The control group returned to ambulation and everyday activities in 10.7 days. The experimental group returned in 4.4 days. For those with a previous history of ankle injury, 16 patients in the control group took an average of 12.0 days to recover, and 18 patients in the experimental group took 4.7 days. For those aspirated and injected, an increased range of motion was noted following aspiration. The injection helped to relieve pain, and even after 30 minutes to an hour, most did not experience as much pain as they did prior to the injection.

Problem: Loss of Motion

As mentioned earlier, swelling results in loss of motion in the ankle joint. Once swelling is under control it is essential to work toward regaining full range of motion through participation in a series of stretching exercises. This must be attained before the patient can engage in the necessary strengthening exercises.

It is important to emphasize that the most common reason for chronic pain and reinjury following an ankle sprain, in our experience, is decreased range of motion, primarily dorsiflexion. The common emergency room plan of crutches, Ace bandage wrap, and "stay off it for awhile" contributes to loss of motion by allowing the foot to be held in a plantar flexed inverted position. This places the foot and ankle in a dependent position without benefit of muscle action to increase venous and lymphatic return, ultimately increasing edema. Edema is a major cause of loss of motion. Early, pain-free ambulation is a significant factor in maintaining normal range of motion. A simple method for determining whether the athlete has decreased motion is as follows: Have the athlete place both feet (without shoes) on the floor, hip width apart and parallel. Next, instruct the athlete to bend both knees and both ankles while keeping the feet flat on the floor. Then, observe for a difference in motion (Fig 3–17,A-C).

Jackson et al.[15] administered a three-phase treatment program to 105 cadets suffering from ankle injuries of different severities in order to assess the relation between severity and the time of total functional recovery. Phase 2 of the three-part treatment protocol consisted of exercises aimed at the restoration of motion. These exercises were performed for 20 minutes, and were preceded by 20 minutes of soaking in a cool whirlpool, and 20 minutes of application of an intermittent pressure stocking. They reported that the total days of disability from date of injury to release to full activity was 8 days for mild injuries, 15 for moderate, and 19 days for severe. They expressed the opinion that what constitutes the "best" treatment program varies according to several different factors, namely, the severity of the injury, the individual's response to injury, and the different performance requirements of each athlete. The authors emphasized that rehabilitation of the ankle should continue beyond taping. Achieving a full painless range of motion is necessary to prevent chronic pain and reinjury.

Vegso and Harmon[25] have reported the importance of dorsiflexion of the ankle joint. They outlined a specific test and exercise program to delineate and control the problem of loss of dorsiflexion.

Range of motion exercises for dorsiflexion may be started within 24 hours, depending on the severity of the injury. This should be done actively or in an active-assisted manner through partial weight-bearing, as shown in Figure 3–18,A. A wedge board (Fig 3–19) may also be used to perform this exercise (Fig 3–18,B). Calf stretching is also permitted as tolerated (Fig 3–20). Plantar flexion, inversion, and eversion should be avoided in the early rehabilitation phase in order to permit adequate soft tissue healing.

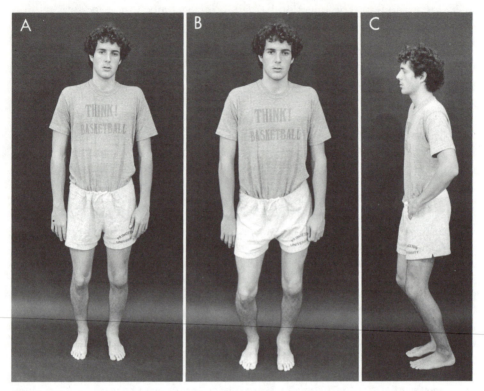

FIG 3–17.
A, in the ankle range-of-motion test, the starting position is with feet parallel and apart to width of hips. **B,** decreased range of motion in ankle is shown. **C,** lateral view.

REHABILITATION: RANGE OF MOTION AND CALF STRETCHING

The procedure for the range-of-motion and flexibility exercises to improve dorsiflexion is as follows:

Range of Motion
Position.—In a standing position, place the injured ankle/leg forward. Toes should be pointed straight ahead. Extend the opposite leg behind.
    Bend the injured ankle and knee. Keep the foot flat on the floor.
    There should be a "stretch" in the ankle and Achilles tendon.
    Hold this stretched position for 10 seconds.
    Repeat this exercise 15 to 20 times, three times a day (see Fig 3–18,A).
    Repeat this exercise with the wedge board (see Fig 3–18,B).

Calf Stretching
Position.—In a standing position, place the injured ankle/leg *behind* the uninjured ankle/leg. Feet should be hip-width apart. Toes should be pointed straight ahead.
    Face a wall for support. Lean forward (hands on the wall), keeping the injured leg straight.

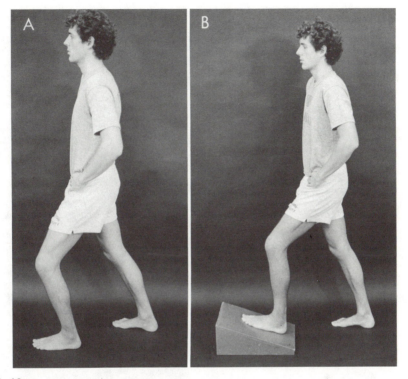

FIG 3–18.
A, ankle range of motion (dorsiflexion) is shown. Left ankle and knee are flexed; foot is flat on the floor. **B,** ankle range of motion on a wedge board (dorsiflexion) is shown. Left ankle and knee are flexed.

>　There should be a "stretch" in the ankle and calf.
>　Hold this stretched position for 10 seconds.
>　Repeat this exercise 15 to 20 times, three times day (see Fig 3–20).

Heelcord Stretch

　The following is a description of the heelcord exercises, both with and without the heelcord box.

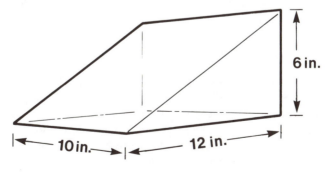

FIG 3–19.
Wedge board made of ½-in. plywood is used as an aid for calf stretching and ankle range-of-motion exercises.

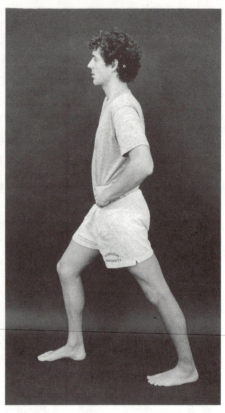

FIG 3–20.
Calf stretching exercise is shown for the left leg.

1. Stand with feet in a parallel position, toes pointing straight ahead, in front of a wall. With both hands on the wall for support, lean forward, keeping both legs straight. There should be a stretch either in the Achilles tendon or in the anterior aspect of the ankle (Fig 3–21,A). Hold this for 6 to 10 seconds. Return to starting position. Repeat 15 to 20 times, two to three times a day.

2. Repeat the above exercise with bent legs. Stand with feet parallel, bend both knees, and then lean forward (Fig 3–21,B).

3. Repeat both of the above exercises using heelcord box (Figs 21,C and D).

Problem: Loss of Strength

The loss of motion that results from swelling in ankle injuries is often accompanied by a loss of strength. Once range of motion has been regained, it is possible to work toward eliminating this deficit. A review of the literature shows that ankle instability and proprioceptive deficit can be attributed to insufficient strength in the peroneal muscles. Strengthening exercises are essential not only as an aid to recovery, but as preventive measure against reinjury.

Glick et al.[12] studied the muscle function of the lower leg. Their testing showed the importance of strong peroneals to support the ankle mortise

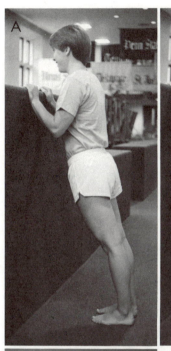
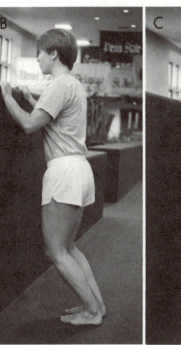
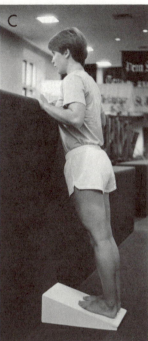

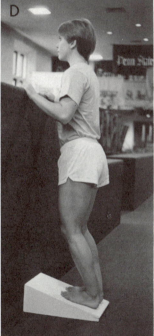

FIG 3–21.
A, ankle range of motion can be regained through heelcord stretching. The position in which the stretch is held is shown; feet are parallel and flat on the floor, and knees are extended. **B,** heelcord stretching can also be done with bent legs. The position in which the stretch is held is shown; the feet remain flat on the floor, and the knees and ankles are flexed. **C,** heelcord stretching can be done with the heelcord box. The exercise in which the legs are extended is shown. **D,** heelcord stretching using the heelcord box in the bent leg position.

in preventing injuries. The necessity for strong peroneals implies the necessity of making strengthening exercises a major part of the rehabilitation program.

Garrick[11] provides a protocol for ankle sprain rehabilitation similar to the one recommended in this chapter.

Jackson et al.[15] recommended ankle strengthening exercises in the third phase of their treatment program. Patients performed toe raises against a Universal gym apparatus and inversion-eversion resistance exercises on an ankle machine.

REHABILITATION: HEEL AND TOE RAISES/WALKING

Toe raises are performed to increase strength in the posterior muscle group. They should be done on a wedge board (Figs 3–22,A and B), stool (Figs 3–23,A and B), or step so that the muscles work through a full range of motion.

Heel and toe walking are also performed to improve muscular strength, endurance, and neuromuscular function. The position of the feet should be

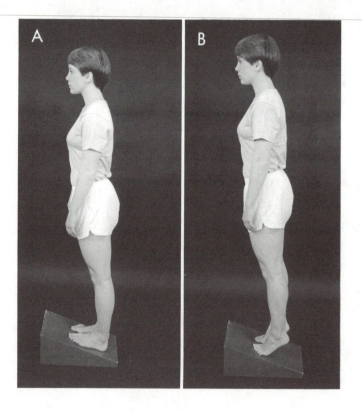

FIG 3–22.
This patient is performing toe raises on a wedge board. **A,** in the starting position, the heels are lower to allow for full range of motion. **B,** end position should be held for 4 to 6 seconds.

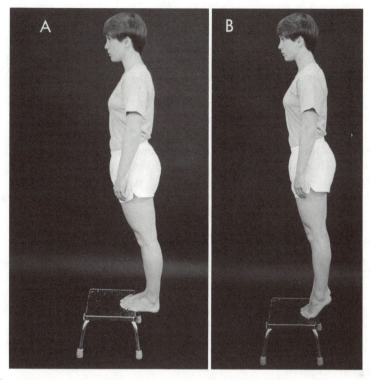

FIG 3–23.
This patient is performing toe raises, using a stool. **A,** in the starting position the heels are lower than the stool to allow for full range of motion strengthening. **B,** end position should be held for 4 to 6 seconds.

changed so that they are inverted or everted while the heel and toe walking are performed.

The toe and heel raises, and walking exercise programs are as follows:

Toe Raises
Position.—Stand on both feet.

Action.—Raise up on the toes of both feet. Hold this position for 4 to 6 seconds. Perform 10 to 20 repetitions. After 30 seconds, perform an additional 10 to 20 repetitions. When it is possible to do the maximum number of repetitions without fatigue, do the toe raises by raising up on the injured foot only.

Toe Walking

Stand on toes and walk as long as possible, up to 5 minutes. Repeat two times per day.

Heel Walking

Walk on heels for as long as possible, up to five minutes. Repeat two times per day. If soreness develops, use *ice* for 20 minutes following each exercise session.

REHABILITATION: "THERABAND"/SURGICAL TUBING

Dorsiflexion, inversion and eversion strength can be increased through the use of surgical tubing, "Theraband," manual resistance, isotonic, isokinetic, or isometric exercises at various angles.

Ankle exercises using "Theraband" or surgical tubing consist of the following:

Eversion (Outward)
Position.—Sit with knees, ankles, and feet together. Attach the "Theraband" around both feet.

Action.—With feet in full dorsiflexion (up), move the front of the feet apart and return. Do 10 to 12 repetitions. With feet in neutral position (90 degrees) move feet apart and return. Do 10 to 12 repetitions (Figs 3–24,A and B).

Inversion (Inward)
Position.—Sit with lower legs and feet crossed and outsides of feet together. Place the "Theraband" around the front of both feet (Fig 3–25,A).

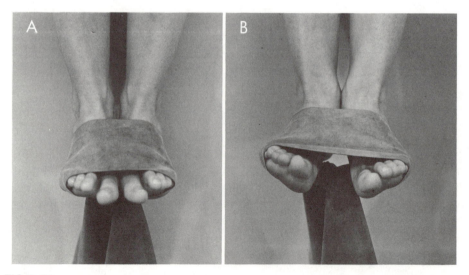

FIG 3–24.
A, eversion strength training can be done with surgical tubing, "Theraband," or a bicycle inner tube. In the starting position the ankles, heels, and first metatarsophalangeal joints are held together and the ankles are dorsiflexed to 90 degrees. **B,** the fully everted position for eversion strength training is shown.

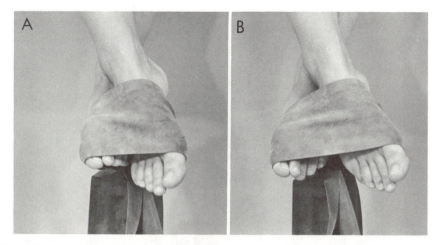

FIG 3–25.
A, for inversion strengthening with "Theraband," in the starting position, the ankles are crossed and "Theraband" is placed around the feet. **B,** the fully inverted position for inversion strengthening is shown.

Action.—Move feet apart and return. Repeat 10 to 15 times. After 30 seconds, repeat 10 to 15 times (Fig 3–25,B).

There are a variety of other methods employed to increase range of motion, strength, and muscular endurance of the ankle.

Although not widely available, the Elgin ankle exerciser (Elgin Exerciser Appliance Co., Sandwich, Ill.) (Fig 3–26) and the Cybex II (Cybex—Division of Lumex Inc., Ronkonkoma, N.Y.) have proved to be extremely effective in rehabilitating ankle injuries.

REHABILITATION: ELGIN ANKLE EXERCISER

An exercise program using the Elgin ankle exerciser is described below:

To Strengthen the Ankle Plantar Flexors
Position.—Begin with the foot in the fully dorsiflexed position (dorsiflexed at 90 degrees). The thigh should not be internally or externally rotated. The weight is placed on the spool closest to the patient (Fig 3–27,A).

Action.—The patient should then plantar flex the foot until it reaches the fully contracted plantar flexed position (Fig 3–27,B). Hold the fully contracted position for 2 seconds. Return to the starting position, and repeat for three sets of 10 to 12 repetitions one to two times a day.

To Strengthen the Ankle Dorsiflexors
Position.—Begin with the foot in the fully plantar flexed position. The weight is placed on the spool farthest from the patient on the vertical axis.

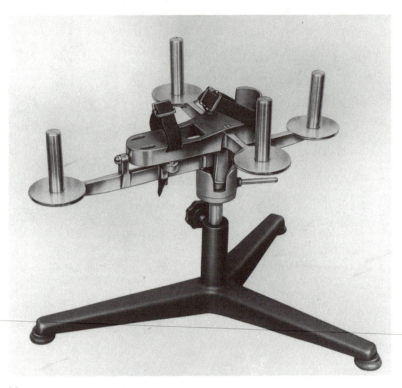

FIG 3–26.
The Elgin ankle exerciser, used for lower leg strengthening of the dorsiflexor and plantar flexor muscles and invertor and evertor muscle groups. (From Elgin Exercise Equipment Corp., Des Plaines, Ill. Used with permission.)

Action.—The patient should then dorsiflex the foot until it reaches the fully contracted dorsiflexed position (Fig 3–28). Hold the fully contracted position for 2 seconds. Return to the starting position, and repeat for three sets of 10 to 12 repetitions one to two times a day.

To Strengthen the Ankle Invertors
Position.—Begin with the ankle in the fully everted position. Again, the knee and thigh should not turn inward, but should remain straight ahead. The weight should be placed on the spool on the medial side (Fig 3–29,A).

Action.—The patient should move the foot through the range of motion until it reaches the fully contracted inverted position (Fig 3–29,B). Hold the fully contracted position for 2 seconds. Return to the initial position and repeat the exercise for three sets of 10 to 12 repetitions one to three times a day.

To Strengthen the Ankle Evertors
Position.—Begin with the ankle in the fully inverted position. The weight should be placed on the spool on the lateral side (Fig 3–30,A).

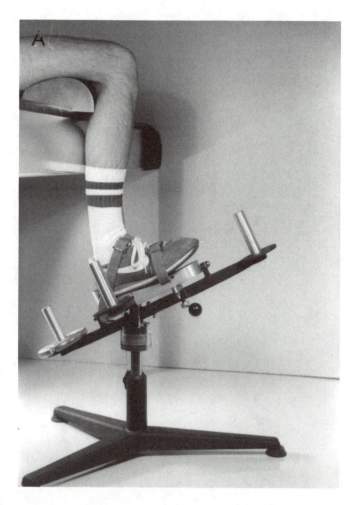

FIG 3–27.
Elgin ankle exercises for strengthening the ankle plantar flexors. **A,** start in the fully dorsiflexed position. (Continued.)

Action.—The patient should move the foot through the range of motion until it reaches the fully contracted everted position (Fig 3–30,B). Return to the initial position and repeat the exercise for three sets of 10 to 12 repetitions, one to two times a day.

Cybex

Isokinetic exercises similar to the ones described above can be performed on the Cybex II (Figs 3–31,A and B). The value and purpose of isokinetic exercises, and their difference from isotonics is discussed in Chapter 1.

The advantage to performing exercises on the Cybex II is that it allows for isolation of specific muscle groups. When plantar and dorsiflexion exercises are done with the knee in full extension (Figs 3–32,A and B), the gastrocnemius,

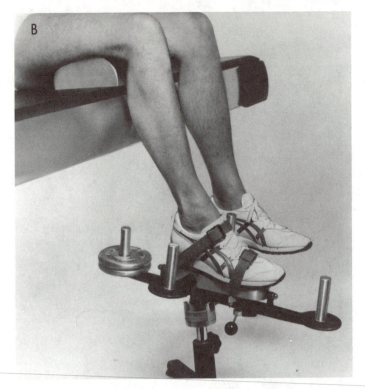

FIG 3–27 (cont.).
B, end in fully contracted plantar flexed position.

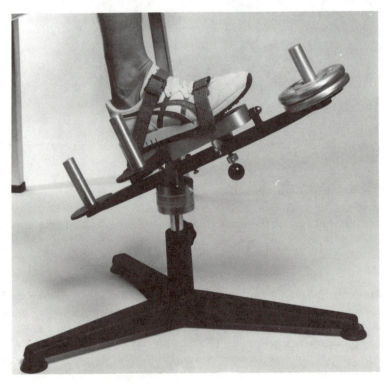

FIG 3–28.
End in the fully contracted, dorsiflexed position.

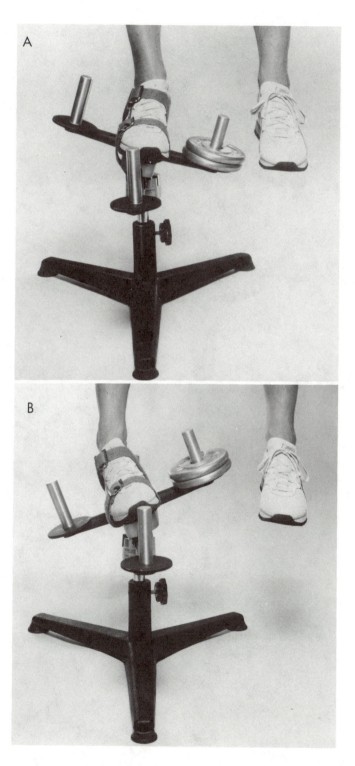

FIG 3–29.
Elgin ankle exercises for strengthening the ankle invertors. **A,** start with the ankle in full eversion. **B,** end in the fully contracted inverted position.

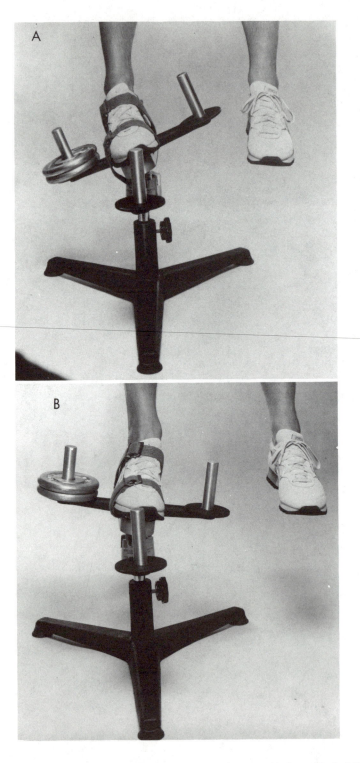

FIG 3–30.
Elgin ankle exercises for strengthening the ankle evertors. **A,** start with the ankle in full inversion.
B, end in the fully contracted, everted position.

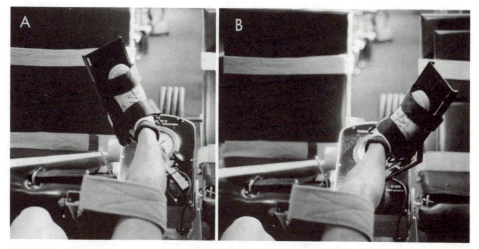

FIG 3–31.
The arrangement for the use of the Cybex to perform exercises to strengthen the invertor and evertor muscle groups. **A,** full inversion is shown. **B,** full eversion is shown.

which originates above the knee, can be isolated. This is the position in which its plantar flexion torque capability is greatest. When these exercises are done with the leg in 90 degrees of knee flexion, the soleus is emphasized (Figs 3–33,A and B).

Problem: Loss of Proprioception

Fiore and Leard[7] and Freeman and others[8–10] emphasize the importance of proprioceptive and neuromuscular function at the ankle joint. This aspect of re-

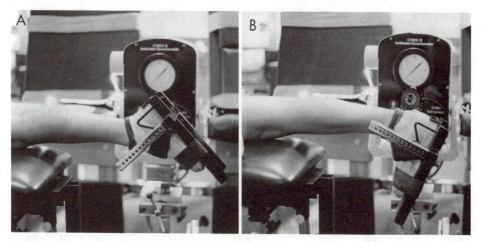

FIG 3–32.
The arrangement for the use of the Cybex to perform exercises to strengthen the dorsi flexor and plantar flexor muscles with the knee in full extension. **A,** the fully plantar flexed position is shown. **B,** the fully dorsiflexed position is shown.

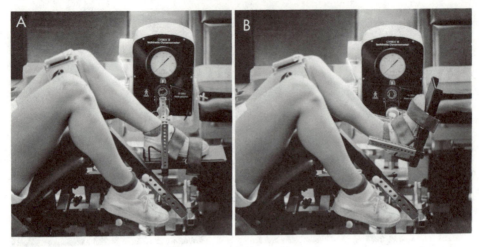

FIG 3–33.
The arrangement for the use of the Cybex to perform exercises to strengthen the dorsiflexor and plantar flexor muscles. The knee is flexed to 90 degrees. **A,** the fully plantar flexed position is shown. **B,** the fully dorsiflexed position is shown.

habilitation is left to chance when the athlete is permitted to return to participation before functional, multiplane, and high-speed activities are incorporated into the rehabilitation program. Allowing this important aspect of rehabilitation to take place in the uncontrolled environment of practice or competition needlessly subjects the athlete to reinjury. Therefore, exercises aimed at restoring proprioceptive and neuromuscular function are recommended.[7–10]

Freeman et al.[8] compared the effect of mobilization and immobilization on the proprioceptive deficits in a group of ankles with ligamentous injuries. Three treatment procedures were compared: (1) immobilization of the foot and ankle, (2) conventional physiotherapy, and (3) mobilization exercises designed to develop coordination. Results showed that treatment consisting of mobilization, namely, coordination exercises, served to both reduce functional instability and proprioceptive deficit to a greater degree than the other two treatment forms. Twelve patients (46%) treated by the other methods complained of the existence of functional instability, as compared to one patient (7%) in the exercise group. Of 13 patients demonstrating a final proprioceptive deficit, only two were in the exercise treatment group.[8]

Fiore and Leard[7] report that the high frequency of ankle and foot injuries can be attributed to the high degree of biomechanical demands and anatomical stresses placed on their individual components. They cite the following statistics from other sources: the ankle and foot receive stresses equivalent to 125% of body weight during walking, 200% while running, and a greater degree of stress in diagonal patterns, from lateral motion. Muscular imbalances and inadequacies in proprioceptive feedback and neuromuscular coordination, while often not apparent, can both affect performance and lead to injury/reinjury. Rehabilitation programs are needed to train, maintain, and "educate" the foot and ankle following injury, and to prepare it for activity. Functional activities alone are needed to bridge the gap that often exists between restoring range of motion and increasing strength and agility. Freeman provides a suggested program, which includes the wobbleboard, Elgin ankle exerciser, heel and toe walking, and "Theraband". The wobbleboard is to improve balance and coordination.[7]

Leach[17] states that the main objective in rehabilitation is to obtain functional return to activity. He calls for immediate mobilization and cites the work of Freeman on proprioception and its importance to the return to activity. He also emphasizes the use of agility exercises, particularly sport-specific exercises, for returning proprioception to normal.[17]

REHABILITATION: AGILITY AND PROPRIOCEPTIVE EXERCISES

It is therefore recommended that activities such as those in the following list should be used to redevelop proprioceptive and neuromuscular functions and to determine the athlete's ability to perform at a level necessary to return to activity safely. The ankle should be supported with adhesive strapping for these activities: (1) heel and toe walking; (2) teeter board; (3) rope-skipping; (4) straight-ahead jogging; (5) straight-ahead running; (6) backward running; (7) running circles (5-yd diameter) (a) clockwise, (b) counterclockwise, and (c) backward and forward; (8) 90 degree cuts while running; (9) running zigzags at 45 degrees; and (10) other sport-specific agility and skill activities.

Below is a recommended agility program:

Warm-up

A quarter to a half mile of easy jogging, eight to ten minutes per mile.

Agility

1. Three to five 10-yd sprints—half speed.
2. Three to five 10-yd sprints—three-quarters speed.
3. Three to five 40-yd sprints—three-quarters speed.
4. Five circles to the right (start with 10-yd diameter circle).
5. Five circles to the left (circle and decrease to 5-yd diameter circle (Fig 3–34).
6. Five to ten figure-of-eight circles (5-yd diameter circle) (Fig 3–35).
7. Five boxes to the right, (5-yd squares) five boxes to the left (Fig 3–36).
8. Five- to 10-yd backward sprints–half speed.
9. Three to five cariocas to the right for 20 yd—half speed; three to five cariocas to the left for 20 yds—half speed (Fig 3–37).
10. One 100-yd sprint—half speed.

Warm-down

A quarter to a half mile of easy jogging—10 minutes per mile.

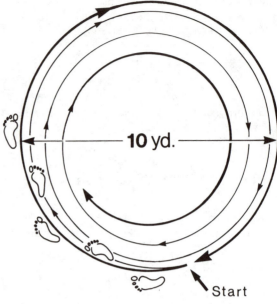

FIG 3–34.
When running circles, the patient should run five circles counterclockwise, beginning with a 10-yd diameter circle. Initially, the patient should run all 10-yd diameter circles, gradually reducing the diameter to no less than 5 yd. The patient should run five clockwise circles as well, using the same procedure.

FIG 3–35.
The patient is to run figure-of-eight patterns according to the diagram at right.

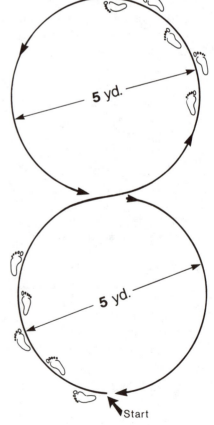

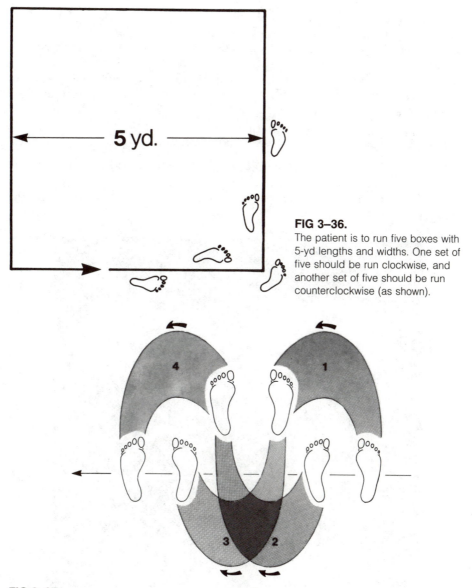

FIG 3–36.
The patient is to run five boxes with 5-yd lengths and widths. One set of five should be run clockwise, and another set of five should be run counterclockwise (as shown).

FIG 3–37.
The patient is to run two sets of three to five cariocas, one moving from left to right, and one from right to left, as shown. When moving from right to left, the patient is to begin by crossing the right leg in front of the left *(step 1)*, and proceed to cross the left behind the right *(step 2)*, the right behind the left *(step 3)*, and the left in front of the right *(step 4)*. The patient should continue this pattern for 20 yds, beginning slowly and gradually increasing to half speed.

REHABILITATION: WOBBLEBOARD

As explained earlier, the wobbleboard is used to improve balance and coordination.

The exercises involving both the unilateral and multidirectional board (Fig 3–38,A and B) implemented at the University of Pennsylvania Sports Medicine Center are described below.

Exercises on the Unidirectional Wobbleboard

For each of the exercises described below, the athlete is instructed to rock back and forth in a controlled manner, three minutes in each direction.

When exercising the injured leg, the patient is to stand on that leg only. Use a wall or chair for support.

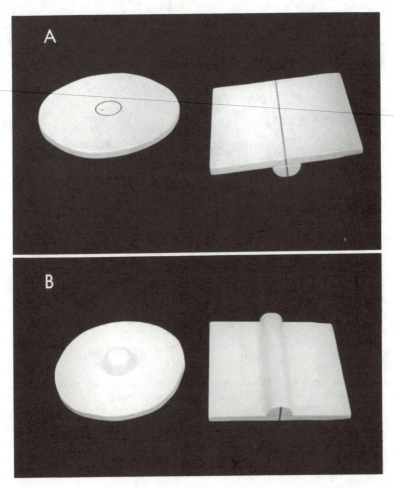

FIG 3–38.
A, the wobbleboard for uniplane, proprioceptive exercises is shown *(right)*. The wobbleboard for multidirectional proprioceptive exercise is also shown *(left)*. **B,** bottom views of the unidirectional *(right)* and multidirectional *(left)* wobbleboards.

Exercises for Plantar Flexion and Dorsiflexion.—Follow the steps given below.

1. Place the injured foot on the wobbleboard with the axis of the board running perpendicular to the foot (Fig 3–39,A).
2. Rock back and forth, touching the front edge of the board to the floor, then touch the back edge to the floor, and so on.

Exercises for Inversion and Eversion.—Follow the steps given below.

1. Place the injured foot on the wobbleboard with the axis of the board running vertical to the foot (Fig 3–39,B).
2. Rock back and forth in a controlled manner, touching the right edge of the board to the floor, and then touch the left edge to the floor, and so on.

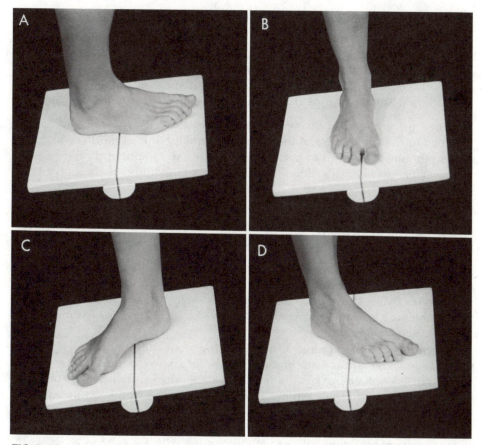

FIG 3–39.
Unidirectional wobbleboard exercises—the patient is instructed to rock back and forth in a controlled manner for up to three minutes in each direction. **A,** the wobbleboard position for plantar flexion and dorsiflexion is shown. **B,** positioning for inversion and eversion. **C,** positioning for pronation and supination at 45 degrees of external rotation. **D,** positioning for pronation and supination at 45 degrees of internal rotation.

Exercises for Supination and Pronation in 45 Degrees External Rotation.—Follow the steps given below.

1. Place the foot on the wobbleboard diagonally, as shown in Figure 3–39,C.
2. Rock back and forth, touching first the right edge of the board to the floor, and then touch the left edge to the floor, and so on.

Exercises for Supination and Pronation at 45 Degrees Internal Rotation.—Follow the steps given below.

1. Place the foot on the wobbleboard diagonally, as shown in Figure 3–39,D.
2. Rock back and forth, touching first the right edge of the board to the floor, and then touch the left edge to the floor, and so on.

Exercises Using the Multidirectional Wobbleboard.—Follow the steps given below.

1. Place the injured foot on the multidirectional board (Fig 3–40,A).
2. Using a wall or chair for support, rotate the ankle clockwise, rolling the edge close to the floor, but not touching it (Fig 3–40,B).
3. Repeat step 2, rotating the ankle in the opposite direction.

Once the athlete is capable of performing all of his or her sport-specific activities to the satisfaction of the physician, athletic trainer, and coach, he or she is permitted to return to participation. Adhesive strapping should be used for participation following injury and it should be continued throughout the season.

Problem: Instability

Ankle instability can be dealt with by combining several different treatment procedures. In addition to the heel and toe walking, "Theraband," Elgin ankle exerciser, and Cybex II exercises described previously, the use of adhesive strapping techniques and the Aircast ankle training brace (Aircast Inc., Summit, N.J.) are to be considered.

Freeman[10] compared three forms of treatment: mobilization, immobilization for six weeks, and suture with immobilization for six weeks, for their respective effects on ankle stability. Results led to the support of mobilization over the other two treatment forms. While stability was observed in the suture-with-immobilization group, the time period in which it took those treated by mobilization to become symptom-free was 12 weeks, approximately half that for those treated by immobilization with or without suture, which was 22 to 26 weeks.[10]

TAPE APPLICATION

Taping[1] is only secondary to a functional rehabilitation program aimed at resolving the inflammation and restoring range of motion, strength, and neuro-

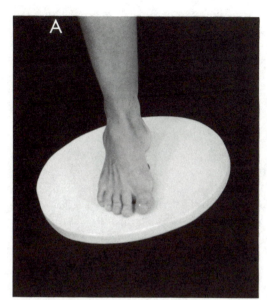

FIG 3–40.
A, multidirectional wobbleboard for proprioceptive exercise. **B,** the foot rolls in a clockwise and counterclockwise direction, without the edge of the board touching on floor. This exercise is to be performed while standing on the injured leg only.

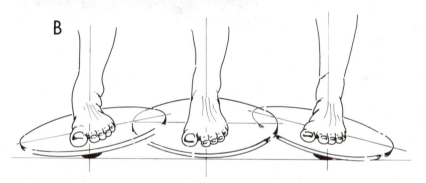

muscular coordination. Used in this context, tape is beneficial in the early stages of rehabilitation for the purposes of immobilization, compression, and support of the affected soft tissues. As the athlete progresses through the various stages of rehabilitation and gradually returns to practice and competition, the tape helps to decrease the likelihood of reinjury.

The use of prophylactic adhesive strappings for selected injuries to the foot, ankle, and lower leg has been readily adopted by orthopedists, athletic trainers, coaches, and others peripherally involved in sports medicine. To justify the use of adhesive strappings, an accurate diagnosis and thorough evaluation of the extent of tissue damage is required. Only then can taping practices be highly effective in supporting and protecting soft tissue structures that have been weakened as a result of acute or chronic injuries.

Adhesive strappings, used in the appropriate circumstances and applied properly, can assist in the process of healing and reconditioning. However, when carelessly and improperly applied, strapping can result in impairment of circulation, discomfort, and aggravation of soft tissue injuries.

The following principles[1] are considered basic to the application of adhesive strapping to the ankle, foot, and lower leg.

1. An understanding of anatomy and biomechanics is necessary. Once the mechanism of injury and the underlying irritated tissues are identified, a decision can be made as to the appropriate adhesive strapping.

2. To receive maximum support and protection from the tape, the joint or irritated area must be positioned in a manner conducive to counteracting the forces that contribute to the initial injury. For example, an inversion plantar-flexion injury to the ankle requires placement of the joint in a neutral position with slight eversion.

3. The area to be taped must be thoroughly cleaned, shaved, and free from the possibility of skin irritation. This predicates the use of protective dressing over abrasions or cuts and other highly sensitive areas. In the latter the tape applied to the ankle can contribute to mechanical irritation of the skin and the distal aspect of the Achilles tendon and the area anterior to the ankle joint. The use of lubricated gauze sponges will help to prevent blistering of the skin in these sensitive areas.

4. The practice of strapping directly to the skin enhances the adhesive qualities of the tape. However, pretaping underwrap is recommended if there will be repeated application and removal of the tape to the same area. The underwrap helps to decrease the possibility of skin breakdown and facilitates the removal of the tape after use.

5. Continuous taping, especially over the areas in which the contour and shape of the extremity changes, tends to result in unequal pressure and can impede normal blood flow. Therefore, it is recommended that the adhesive strapping be applied in strips. If each strip overlaps the preceding one by a half to three-quarters, more equal pressure can be attained and separation of the tape during strenuous activity can be prevented.

6. To further prevent impairment of circulation and restriction of motion, caution should be exercised in encircling the tape around a muscle belly mass. If encircling the muscle is required, as in an Achilles tendon strapping, elastic tape should be used because of its expansive properties.

7. To prevent gapping of the tape, the proper size should be selected. For areas of the foot, a width of 1 in. allows for the greatest ease of application, whereas the ankle joint requires tape 1½ in. wide.

8. An adhesive strapping should be removed promptly after a practice session or athletic contest. In all other circumstances, it should not be left on for more than three days. After removal of the tape, the skin should be cleansed with alcohol, powdered, and prepared for reapplication of the tape if necessary.[2]

CONCLUSION

It is difficult and unwise to put time constraints on the rate of recovery or specific aspects of recovery. One may find that an athlete who suffers from a grade I inversion sprain will progress through the entire rehabilitation program in three days; conversely, a nonsurgical grade III or greater inversion sprain may take up to eight weeks before complete recovery is achieved. It would seem, therefore, that a combination would be appropriate. Emphasis should be placed on early and continued use of ice, the return to full range of motion and strength, and the inclusion of activities designed to reintegrate neuromuscular function.

REFERENCES

1. Bonci CM: Adhesive strapping techniques. *Clin Sports Med* 1982; 1:99–116.
2. Brady TA, Arnold A: Aspiration injection treatment for varus sprain of the ankle: A preliminary report. *J Bone Joint Surg Am* 1972; 54:1257–1261.
3. Brostrom L: Sprained ankles: V. Treatment and prognosis in recent ligament ruptures. *Acta Chir Scand* 1966; 132:537.
4. Brown A: Physical medicine in rehabilitation. *Md Med J* 1970; 19:61.
5. Dameron TB: Management of acute ankle sprains. *South Med J* 1977; 70:1166.
6. Eitner D: Uses of heat, in Kuprian W (ed): *Physical Therapy for Sports*. Philadelphia, WB Saunders Co, 1982, pp 52–61.
7. Fiore RD, Leard JS: Functional approach in the rehabilitation of the ankle and rear foot. *Athletic Training*, Winter 1980, pp 231–235.
8. Freeman MAR, Dean MRE, Hanham IWF: The etiology and prevention of functional instability of the foot. *J Bone Joint Surg Br* 1965; 47:678–685.
9. Freeman MAR: Instability of the foot after injuries to the lateral ligaments of the ankle. *J Bone Joint Surg Br* 1965; 47:669–677.
10. Freeman MAR: Treatment of ruptures of the lateral ligament of the ankle. *J Bone Joint Surg Br* 1965; 47:661–668.
11. Garrick JG: 'When can I . . . ?'—a practical approach to rehabilitation illustrated by treatment of ankle injury. *Am J Sports Med* 1981; 9(1):67–68.
12. Glick JM, Gordon RB, Nishimoto D: The prevention and treatment of ankle injuries. *Am J Sports Med* 1976; 4(4):136–141.
13. Gucker T: Heat and cold in orthopedics, in Licht S (ed): *Therapeutic Heat and Cold*. Baltimore, Waverly Press Inc, 1965, pp 398–406.
14. Hocutt JE, Jaffe R, Rylander CR, et al: Cryotherapy in ankle sprains. *Am J Sports Med* 1982; 10(5):316–319.
15. Jackson DW, Ashley RL, Powell JW: Ankle sprains in young athletes. *Clin Orthop* 1974; 101:201–215.
16. Kalenak A, et al: Athletic injuries: Heat vs. cold. *Am Fam Physician* 1975; 12:131–135.
17. Leach RE: The prevention and rehabilitation of soft tissue injuries. *Int J Sports Med* 1982; 3:18–20.
18. Licht S (ed): *Therapeutic Heat and Cold*. Baltimore, Waverly Press Inc, 1965.
19. McCluskey GM, Blackburn TA, Lewis T: A treatment for ankle sprains. *Am J Sports Med* 1976; 4:158.
20. McMaster WC: A literary review of ice therapy on injuries. *Am J Sports Med* 1977; 5:124.
21. Millard JB: Conductive heating, in Licht S (ed): *Therapeutic Heat and Cold*. Baltimore, Waverly Press Inc, 1965.
22. Starkey JA: Treatment of ankle sprains by simultaneous use of intermittent compression and ice packs. *Am J Sports Med* 1976; 4(4):142–144.
23. Stilwell GK: General principles in thermotherapy, in Licht S (ed): *Therapeutic Heat and Cold*. Baltimore, Waverly Press Inc, 1965.

24. Stover CN: Air-Stirrup management of ankle injuries in the athlete. *Am J Sports Med* 1980; 8(5):360–365.
25. Vegso JJ, Harmon LE: Nonoperative management of athletic ankle injuries. *Clin Sports Med* 1982; 1:85–97.
26. Zoltan JD: Treatment of ankle sprains with joint aspiration, xylocaine, infiltration, and early mobilization. *J Trauma* 1977; 17:93–96.

CHAPTER 4

The Leg

INJURY: 'SHIN SPLINTS'
Problem: Pain

There is a lack of agreement among physicians concerning the clinical entity commonly known as "shin splints." There is disagreement over the anatomical location of the injury, its etiology, and the typical clinical course.[8] While this term has been used to refer to leg pain, it should in fact be discussed as six specific diagnoses. Jackson provides such a classification scheme, which is cited by Andrews as well.[1, 8]

The specific diagnoses that should be used in assessing the injuries are: (1) musculotendinous inflammation (tendinitis); (2) musculotendinous tear (strain); (3) stress fracture of the tibia or fibula; (4) stress reaction of bone; (5) muscle-bone insertion injury; and (6) vascular disorders (compartment syndromes).

The location of pain experienced in the lower leg needs to be differentiated. Its presence anteriorly, posteriorly, medially, or laterally, and identification of which third of the tibia it occurs in, are specifics to be attended to.[8]

For runners logging more than 30 miles a week, the most common shin pain is found "just distal to the muscle insertion on the posterior medial tibia, approximately 10 cm to 15 cm proximal to the tip of the medial malleolus."[8]

The pain characterizing the injury, whether located in the bone, muscle, or tendon, can serve as an indicator for differentiating musculotendinous inflammation and tears from stress reactions and fractures. Both inflammation and tears of the musculotendinous unit are associated with an increase in pain with motion of the toe, foot, and ankle. On the other hand, injuries to the bone are characterized by an increase in pain with weight-bearing.[8] Andrews[1] states that most overuse injuries are associated with running, and cites James' report that out of 232 running injuries, 13% included posterior tibial syndromes, or what is commonly known as "shin splints." Progressing too rapidly in training is a predominant factor contributing to the development of shin splints.[8] In addition to using the classification of shin splints outlined above, Andrews[1] and Eggold[5] distinguish between the anterior and the posterior shin splints.[1]

ANTERIOR SHIN SPLINT SYNDROME

The "anterior shin splint syndrome" involves the irritation and inflammation through overuse of the tibialis anterior, the extensor hallucis and longus, and the extensor digitorum longus. These muscles are involved in several phases of the running gait. The tibialis anterior, specifically, works as a decelerator during the heel strike phase, and to prevent "foot slap" during the midstance phase.[1] Hard heels, hard running surfaces, or forefoot malignment can all be contributing factors.[13] The pain, tenderness, and tightness is felt along the lateral border of the tibia and at the distal third of the tibia along the medial crest. Active dorsiflexion and passive plantar flexion of the ankle will increase the pain.[1, 13]

POSTERIOR SHIN SPLINT SYNDROME

Different muscles that are active after heel contact during the running gait can also becomed inflamed, and this condition is referred to by Andrews as the "posterior shin splint syndrome." The posterior tibialis longus, flexor digitorum longus, and flexor hallucis longus become inflamed from prolonged or abnormal pronation.[1]

The most common injury of the shin splint diagnosis is that of the fatigue tear of the fibers of the posterior tibialis muscle at its insertion into the periostium of the tibia. An anatomical deviation such as foot pronation,[1, 5] and change of surface structure are factors that can contribute to the development of shin splints.[1] Pain can be attributed to the inflammatory edema and myotatic contraction of muscle.

Shoe corrections and improvements are very important in the case of anterior and posterior shin splints. Andrews[1] mentions the necessity of using shoes with a sole that allows for more shock absorption, and the effective use of orthotics, as does Jackson.[8, 9] A well-fitting heel counter, heel lifts,[13] heel cushions, and shoes with adequate foreflex[13] are also effective. Orthotics serve to limit pronation of the subtalar joint.[5, 13, 28, 29] The production, use, and function of orthotics are discussed in Chapter 2.

Abstention from athletic activity is an unpopular, yet effective method for relieving the pain that characterizes shin splints. It should be followed with graduated return to a pain-free activity level.[1, 8–10]

Cryotherapy can be applied in cases of anterior shin splints to reduce the swelling that occurs.[13] It is also effective for treating the inflammation along the crest of the tibia.[8, 9] Acute cases can be iced for 10 to 15 minutes, or until numbing occurs.[1, 13, 23]

The low Dye technique can be applied in cases of shin splints. It acts to correct biomechanical dysfunction. The application procedure and illustrations (see Figs 2–1 through 2–5) can be found in Chapter 2.

Problem: Decreased Flexibility

The inflammation of the tibialis muscles and the flexor and extensor hallucis and longus result in tightness and decreased flexibility.

REHABILITATION: STRETCHING

Stretching is recommended by a variety of authors for the treatment of shin splints. For both the anterior and posterior shin splint syndrome, Andrews recommends stretching of the involved muscle groups and range of motion exercises. Jackson and Kulund state that stretching should be a part of the training program. Kulund's program consists of heelcord stretching with the heelcord box for five minutes, three times a day.[1, 13]

The heelcord exercises should be done 15 times each, two to three times a day. The stretch should be felt in the ankle and calf for the straight leg position, and in the ankle and Achilles tendon in the bent leg position. The stretch should be held for 10 seconds. (Refer to Figs 2–11,A-D, for these exercises.)

The stretching program is outlined following the discussion of stress fractures and stress reactions later in this chapter.

Problem: Decreased Strength

The experience of pain, immobilization of the athlete, or decrease in activity are all factors that contribute to a decrease of strength.

REHABILITATION: STRENGTH TRAINING

Strengthening is recommended as part of the rehabilitation program for shin splints by Andrews, Jackson, and Kulund. Kulund advocates strengthening the anterior muscle groups.[1, 13] Jackson warns against developing muscle imbalances.[8] Kulund recommends dorsiflexing the ankle against a weight sleeve placed over the foot.[13] The program can begin with three repetitions of 2.5 lb and progress to three sets of 10 lb. He also advocates the use of surgical tubing to develop anterior tibial and peroneal strength.

Strengthening exercises include toe raises, heel and toe walking, and "Theraband" exercises. These are described following the section on stress fractures and stress reactions.

INJURY: STRESS FRACTURE

The symptom characterizing stress fracture is a persistent ill-defined sensation of pain in the lower extremity. These injuries, which can involve the femoral neck, patella, proximal or distal tibia, fibula, and the metatarsal bones, are usually incurred by poorly conditioned and novice athletes.[1, 8] Stress fractures are often due to training too rapidly,[8] making alterations, such as changing running speeds or surfaces,[12, 13] and to biomechanical problems as well. Stress fractures to the tibia are found in individuals with cavus feet, while pronated feet can lead to the development of fibular stress fractures.[13] In the 1981 study of Taunton et al.,[30] of 62 runners, a major cause for stress fractures was found to be training intensity. Rapid commencement of training accounted for 27% of the cases and sudden exposure to hills accounted for 6%. Ten percent of the group sustained stress fractures after one severe session, 8% sustained the injury after a rapid increase in mileage, 5% were from using faulty footwear, and 44% were due to a combination of training errors and changes in footwear. Taunton et al. also found that varus alignment of the foot, which leads to prolonged pronation, increased tibial torque, and biomechanical stress, was present in practically all of the athletes.[30] Excessive stress placed on the bones too quickly does not permit for accommodation to the overload. Often, the remodeling that takes place can be painful.[8]

Early diagnoses can be made via bone scans.[13] Treatment consists of rest precluding the activity that was responsible for the injury for approximately eight weeks from when the pain began. Sometimes this healing period can take up to 12 weeks. Roentgenograms can be used to monitor healing. In certain cases involving the tarsal navicular and the base of the fifth metatarsal, cast immobilization is warranted to effect adequate healing.[1] Cryotherapy can help relieve the pain that characterizes these injuries.

Stress fractures, like shin splints, can be treated with the low Dye strapping technique. It provides biomechanical support if the fracture is from a biomechanical source (see Figs 2–1 through 2–5).

INJURY: STRESS REACTIONS

Stress reactions of bone are atypical stress fractures, most often incurred from overuse, and can be detected with bone scans, on which the bone shows a longitudinal bone stress pattern.[1,8] The pain associated with stress reactions is attributed to the rapid bone turnover and remodeling,[8] and the pattern is more characteristic than that which typifies a stress fracture. It increases with direct pressure on the bone and weight-bearing, and is relieved with rest.[1] Andrews,[1] and Jackson and Bailey[9] have provided a detailed description of the pain experienced by 26 athletes with stress reaction injury.

The biomechanical problems that contribute to the development of stress reactions, stress fractures, and other overuse injuries can be corrected with the use of orthotics. The purpose of the orthotic device is to maintain the neutral position of the foot and allow for normal joint function, while preventing excessive inefficient compensatory motions, such as pronation and supination.[5,12] Extensive and prolonged pronation can contribute to the injury.[28,29] Taunton et al.[30] and Eggold[5] favor their use. Proper training, proper conditioning, and proper foot functioning are the three principal factors that can work to prevent or reduce overuse injuries attained through overstress. Subotnick[28,29] focuses on the third factor, and discusses the relationship between proper foot function, which encompasses shoes, stride, and orthotic control of pronation, with the overuse syndromes. Different types of orthotics are required by different types of runners. Flexible supports are said to be preferred for speeds below a 5-min/mile pace, and for middle-distance runners. More rigid, functional supports are required for longer distances and nonathletic use. Subotnick reports that these are well tolerated by about 90% of his patients. Often, a pair of each kind of orthotic is required.[28, 29] (See Figs 2–6 through 2–10.)

REHABILITATION: CALF STRETCHING AND RANGE OF MOTION

As with other injuries to the foot and ankle, return to activity should be accompanied by exercises to stretch the calf and improve the range of motion. The exercises are described below.

Calf Stretching

1. Stand with feet in parallel position, toes pointing straight ahead, in front of wall. With both hands on the wall for support, lean forward, keeping both legs straight. There should be a "stretch" either in the Achilles tendon or in the anterior aspect of the ankle (see Fig 3–21,A). Hold this for 6 to 10 seconds. Return to starting position. Repeat 15 to 20 times, two to three times a day.

2. Repeat the above exercise with bent legs. Stand with feet parallel, bend both knees, and then lean forward (see Fig 3–21,B).

3. Repeat both of the above exercises using the heelcord box (see Figs 3–21,C and D).

STRENGTHENING

Toe raises should be done on a wedge board (see Figs 3–22,A and B), or stool (see instructions in Chapter 3 and Figs 3–23,A and B) so that the muscles work through the full range of motion. The raised position should be held for 4 to 6 seconds. Two sets of 10 to 20 repetitions, with 30 seconds in between the two sets, should be done two times a day. When the maximum number of repetitions can be done without fatigue, the toe raises can be performed on the injured leg only.

Heel and toe walking are also performed to improve muscular strength, endurance, and neuromuscular function. The position of the feet should be changed so that they are inverted and everted while the heel and toe walking are performed. For toe walking, stand on the toes and walk for as long as possible up to five minutes. Repeat two times per day. For heel walking, walk on the heels for as long as possible, up to five minutes. Repeat two times per day. If soreness develops, use ice for 20 minutes following each exercise session.

"Theraband"

Strength can also be improved through the use of "Theraband."

Eversion (Outward).—Follow the steps below.

1. Sit with knees, ankles, and feet together. Attach "Theraband" around both feet.

2. With feet in full dorsiflexion (up), move the front of the feet apart and return. Do 10 to 12 repetitions. With feet in neutral position (90 degrees) move feet apart and return. Do 10 to 12 repetitions (see Figs 3–24,A and B).

Inversion (Inward).—Follow the steps below.

1. Sit with lower legs and feet crossed and outsides of feet together. Place "Theraband" around the front of both feet (see Fig 3–25,A).

2. Move feet apart and hold for 2 seconds. Relax and rest for 30 seconds. Repeat 10 to 15 times (see Fig 3–25,B).

PREVENTION

Certain steps can be taken to help prevent shin splints. Among these are avoiding excessive early training, wearing properly fitted and cushioned athletic shoes, and allowing sufficient time to accommodate to new surfaces and environments. Stretching should be a part of training and running programs. Additional preventive measures that can be taken are monitoring foot structure and lower extremity alignment, and preventing muscle imbalances.

INJURY: ACHILLES TENDINITIS, TENOSYNOVITIS
Problem: Pain/Swelling

In a study by James et al.,[11] Achilles tendinitis accounts for 11% of the complaints from 232 runners, making it the third most common injury in that particular group.[11, 16, 26] Different pathological conditions can cause Achilles tendon pain. True tendinitis involves the inflammation of the Achilles tendon itself.[16] Tenosynovitis is often confused with tendinitis, but it differs in that it is the inflammation of the tendon sheath and mesotendon.[16, 26] Tenderness directly over the tendon, thickening of the tendon or peritendinous tissue, and soft tissue swelling are the physical findings that characterize these injuries.[16] Turco briefly discusses the mechanism behind tenosynovitis, its symptoms, and the treatment procedure.[31] Tenosynovitis is usually caused by direct blows, shoe irritation, overuse, or overstretch. It is characterized by tenderness, swelling, and, sometimes, crepitus.

INJURY: ACHILLES TENDINITIS

Shields[23] discusses the symptoms and treatment of Achilles tendinitis. An aching sensation in the morning, along with tenderness in the area from the muscle belly to the os calcis, and crepitation during plantar and dorsiflexion are the symptoms characterizing the injury.[23] Clancy[4] reports observing the following symptoms: pain above the superior lip of the calcaneous, which presents itself during running and sometimes during walking; crepitus; and local tenderness.

Smart et al.[26] review the etiological mechanisms involved in Achilles tendinitis. The biomechanical factor that he designates is that of prolonged pronation.[5, 26] Slow-motion, high-speed cinematography has enabled researchers to identify that a whipping action or bowstring effect of the Achilles tendon is produced by prolonged pronation, and that this possibly could produce micro-tears. It has been speculated that degenerative changes of the tendon are related to torsional forces transmitted through the tendon during pronation. Orthotics work to shorten the phase of pronation during the support phase of running. Other etiological mechanisms discussed are poorly designed foot-wear, training surfaces, training intensity, poor lower leg flexibility, overuse through excessive mileage, inactivity, local steroid injections, rheumatic conditions, and indirect trauma.[26] Kulund cites changes in shoes and such biomechanical problems as cavus foot as factors that can contribute to the development of Achilles tendinitis.[13] He states that degeneration of the tendon and the formation of granulation tissue occurs about 3.75 cm above the insertion to the os calcis.

Clancy et al.[3] reviewed the literature pertaining to the relationship between Achilles tendinitis and partial rupture. He reported five cases of Achilles tendinitis and compares two cases of subacute Achilles tendinitis to three cases of chronic Achilles tendinitis. Cases lasting less than two weeks were viewed as acute, those lasting between three and six weeks as subacute, and those lasting longer than six weeks as chronic. Pain and tenderness are two symptoms that distinguish one type from another. While pain in acute injuries is present only with prolonged running and decreases with rest, in the subacute stage it is present on initiation of running and increases with sprinting. Tenderness in acute injuries is only found in a small area, while in chronic injuries this area is larger. The subacute phase is also occasionally characterized by crepitus when the foot is plantar flexed or dorsiflexed.[3]

Relief can be attained by refraining from exercise and athletic activities.[12, 23, 26] For acute Achilles tendinitis, Clancy et al.[3, 4] recommend two weeks of rest, in combination with other conservative treatment measures. Leach et al.[16] recommend decreasing mileage. If palpation is pain free after this, then gradual running may be resumed. If not, then Clancy advocates that conservative treatment be continued for a total of six to eight weeks. If relief is not achieved, then surgery is necessary.[3] He also states that chronic tendinitis can be treated conservatively, but that surgery may be required if conservative treatment is not successful after four to six months.[4] The treatment recommended for peritendinitis and peritendinitis with tendinosis consists of withdrawal from activities that promote the symptoms, and may require non–weight-bearing with crutches, or reduced mileage.[26] However, it is again important to emphasize that rest is not a method of treatment that is used exclusively. Addressing the cause of the injury is essential for permanent relief.

For tendinitis, Leach et al.[16] prescribe cryotherapy after exercise. For peritendinitis and peritendinitis with tendinosis, Smart et al.[26] favor an ice massage. They also recommend it before and after exercises in the case of partial ruptures.[26] Kulund recommends cryotherapy for partial ruptures.[13]

Anti-inflammatory medications can be prescribed for tendinitis.[4, 12, 23, 36] Nonsteroidal anti-inflammatory medications are recommended by Shields.[23] Leach et al.[16] advocate the use of phenylbutazone (Butazolidin). Anti-inflammatory agents can also be used to treat peritendinitis with tendinosis. A thorough discussion of anti-inflammatory, steroidal, and other relevant medications can be found in Chapter 12.

Leach et al.[16] recommend immobilization of the leg and foot in a short-leg walking cast for ten days for Achilles tendinitis when there is either acute pain or a chronic injury. According to Shields,[23] conservative treatment for Achilles tendinitis, rest, anti-inflammatory drugs, heel lifts, orthotics, stretching will be successful 80% of the time. When conservative treatment does not alleviate the pain, immobilization in a short-leg cast in an equinus position for three weeks is recommended.[23] If after six months these methods have failed, then surgery may be required. According to Shields, 70% of the patients treated surgically are able to return to their former level of activity.[23]

Tenosynovitis can be treated with shoe correction[4, 12, 16, 23, 31] and tendinitis with heel elevation.[4] Heel lifts act to shorten the tendon and to relieve the "over-stretch" placed on the tendon.

Problem: Decreased Flexibility
REHABILITATION: STRETCHING

Calf stretching exercises are recommended for tendinitis.[12, 16] Leach states that stretching the posterior ankle capsule and the triceps-surae-Achilles complex is a very important part of the conservative treatment procedure[16] (see Figs 2–11,A-D, 3–20, and 3–21). The instructions for this exercise are included earlier in this chapter following the discussion of stress fractures and stress reactions.

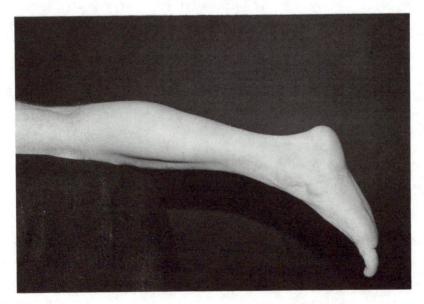

FIG 4–1.
The foot is in the equinus position for strapping of the Achilles tendon.

Adhesive Strapping

This taping procedure[2] is recommended for strains of the Achilles tendon to prevent overstretching of the heelcord through restriction of range of motion in dorsiflexion.

Positioning.—The foot is placed in the equinus position (Fig 4–1).

Materials.—The materials required are 3-in. elastic tape, underwrap, and lubricating gel. Before the application of the tape, the distal aspect of the Achilles tendon should be lubricated to decrease the possibility of mechanical irritation of the skin.

Instructions.—*Step 1.*—Application of the tape begins with two anchor strips. One strip encircles the muscle belly of the gastrocnemius-soleus group, and the other encircles the foot just proximal to the metatarsal heads (Fig 4–2).

Step 2.—A posterior strip is then placed along the length of the Achilles tendon, beginning and ending at the foot and calf anchors, respectively. Before application of this strip, the proximal and distal ends of the tape are split down the middle. The amount of tape split should not exceed the length necessary to completely encircle the foot and calf. The strip is then applied by securing the distal ends of the tape around the foot, pulling upward with firm tension toward the calf, then securing the proximal ends around the muscle belly of the calf group. Depending on the size of the foot, one or two additional posterior strips are applied in the same manner (Fig 4–3).

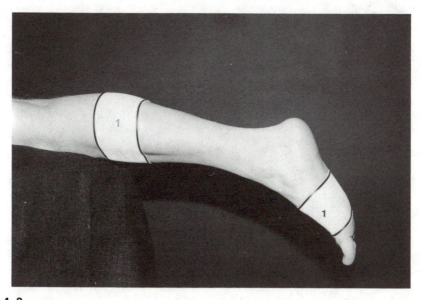

FIG 4–2.
Achilles tendon strapping begins with the application of two anchor strips *(step 1)*.

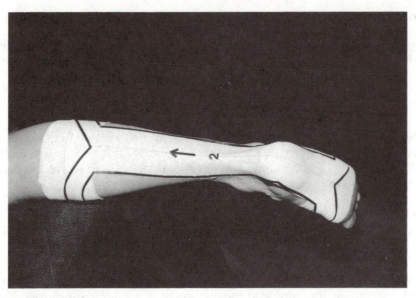

FIG 4–3.
In *step 2*, a posterior strip is placed along the length of the Achilles tendon.

Step 3.—The close-off procedure begins by encircling elastic tape from the metatarsal heads to the calf anchors (Fig 4–4). A pretaping underwrap can be applied before the close-off procedure.[2] Kulund recommends strapping for partial ruptures to the Achilles tendon.[13]

REHABILITATION: STRENGTHENING

Toe raises, as described following the discussion of stress reactions, should be done 10 to 20 times, 2-3 times a day (see Figs 3–22,A and B and 3–23,A and B). Heel and toe walking exercises, also previously described, should be done as well.

Surgery is necessary for those who do not attain relief through conservative measures.[16]

INJURY: ACHILLES TENDON RUPTURE

When stress is placed on the contracted musculotendinous unit where the Achilles tendon conjoins with the gastrocnemius and soleus complex, a rupture of the Achilles tendon can occur. Sudden dorsiflexion can also lead to rupture. Swelling and a gap in the tendon are usually observed. The onset and symptoms of partial Achilles ruptures differ from those of tendinitis and complete rupture. With partial ruptures, there is an acute episode of tearing or snapping, followed by limping and pain.[23] The response to the Thompson test is negative; that is, squeezing the calf causes the foot to plantar flex.[13, 23] In complete ruptures, the response to the Thompson test is positive; these ruptures are usually

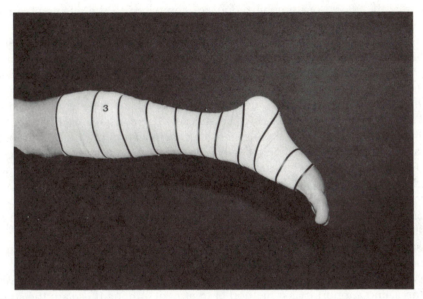

FIG 4–4.
The close-off procedure for this technique is shown.

sustained both by persons who have had chronic symptoms and by those who have had none.[23] The tenderness that characterizes partial ruptures is localized initially, but later becomes more diffuse.[23] Shields[23] relates the occurrence of Achilles ruptures to the degenerative aging process. Clancy et al.[3] describe in detail the clinical course for the five cases of Achilles tendinitis in runners. In their discussion they explain that observations made during microscopic examination indicate that ruptured tendons may not have been normal at the time of injury, and cites literature that supports these observations. Clancy et al.[3] support the viewpoint that the blood supply to the Achilles tendon does not arrive via the musculotendinous unit, but instead through the mesotendineum, and that the development of ruptures is related to the vascular supply to the tendon. They also present a hypothesis for the development of ruptures and cite supportive literature. The hypothesis is that fibroblasts become incapable of synthesizing collagen due to the inflammation that results from the breakdown of the collagen fibril that is brought about by mechanical stress.[3] Achilles tendon ruptures are mostly seen in individuals over 30 years of age. Lessened blood flow can lead to degenerative changes in the tendon.[13] In young, full-grown athletes at the highest level of performance, partial ruptures can occur when training loads are increased.

Problem: Decreased Function

The use of plaster immobilization as a treatment for Achilles tendon injuries is somewhat controversial. In the discussion of the treatment of the ankle, the effects of mobilization were compared with those of immobilization, and arguments were made in favor of one or the other. In the case of Achilles tendon ruptures, the effects of immobilization are compared to the effects of surgical treatment.

Prior to 1968, the approach to treating Achilles tendon ruptures was surgical. This came into question when Lea and Smith[15] presented eight cases in which conservative treatment of Achilles tendon ruptures proved successful. While the accepted approach to tendon ruptures had been surgical, Lea and Smith supported nonoperative treatment, and cited the regenerative ability of the Achilles tendon as the basis for its success. The conservative treatment implemented by Lea and Smith consisted of immobilization of the leg and foot in a gravity equinus walking boot. There was no plantar flexion force applied to the foot. The subjects were immobilized for a period of eight weeks, during which they progressed gradually to weight-bearing. After cast removal they were placed on crutches with a 1-in. heel elevation for full weight-bearing, which was usually after four weeks. Treatment also involved soaks and exercises. Lea and Smith[15] reported that full activity was attained after 16 weeks, and full weight-bearing in a toe-walking gait after 24 weeks. Only one case presented complications and this involved a complete open laceration of the tendon.[15]

Additional studies assess the effect of immobilization on Achilles tendon ruptures, and support it as a method of treatment. Among these are the studies by Gillies and Chalmers,[6] Lea and Smith,[14] Stein and Luekens,[27] Lildholdt and Munch-Jørgensen,[17] and Nistor.[18] These studies utilized a method the same as or similar to that used by Lea and Smith in 1968, and concluded, based on their results, that immobilization is an effective alternative to surgical treatment.

The occurrence of rerupture following treatment and the length of immobilization are two issues of concern. Nistor[19] reviews the reports of rerupture in studies involving conservative treatment. Based on the number of reruptures in the reports by Gillies and Chalmers,[6] Lea and Smith,[14, 15] and Inglis et al.,[7] Nistor reports that the overall percentage for reruptures was somewhat less than 10%. Several studies have reported a high incidence of reruptures when Achilles tendons are treated conservatively. The average was 10% but 22% was reported by Jacobs et al.,[10] and 39% by Inglis et al,[7] and Nistor reports the highest incidence of rerupture to be 35%.[19] It is important to remember that comparisons should be made with the amount of complications in the surgically treated cases. Among the complications to be considered are wound infection, skin necrosis, and fistula formation.[19] Immobilization is recommended not only because it yields successful results, but because it eliminates some of the complications and hazards that have been observed in operative cases. In the study by Lea and Smith,[14] for surgical cases, one out of every 5.8 cases (17%) involved major complications.[14, 19]

The length of immobilization is considered to be important. In their 1972 study of 66 cases, Lea and Smith[14] reported seven cases of reruptures; four of these were in patients who were only immobilized for six weeks. This was cited as support for an eight-week immobilization period.[14] Nistor also discusses the possibility that the incidence of rerupture in conservatively treated cases could be decreased if the period of immobilization was lengthened.[19] The regenerative ability of the Achilles tendon is cited as the basis for the success of immobilization.[15]

Other studies compared the results of immobilization to the results of surgical treatment.[10, 19, 25] While Jacobs et al.[10] advocate operative over conservative treatment, Skeoch[25] concludes that conservative care is justifiable for partial subcutaneous Achilles tendon ruptures, but that if it does not prove successful by six months after implementation, a surgical approach is warranted.[25] Smart et al.[26] recommend rest and symptomatic treatment for partial ruptures and surgical repair for small ruptures whose symptoms persist. He advocates conservative treatment when the postoperative risks outweigh the surgical benefits, or when maximal reattainment of tendon function is not essential.[26]

Surgical treatment of chronic partial ruptures is necessary when five to six months of conservative treatment have not been successful.[23] Surgery should consist of surgical excision of the necrotic tendon and reconstruction with a fascial graft. Surgery is also recommended for the treatment of acute ruptures.[23] Research has demonstrated that surgical repair yields stronger tendons than conservative treatment.[7, 23] Inglis et al.,[7] unlike the many who advocate conservative treatment, support surgical treatment. According to the results of their study, both the subjective and the objective functional results were more satisfactory for those treated surgically than those treated nonsurgically. Out of the 44 patients treated surgically, there were two wound infections but no reruptures. Out of 23 nonsurgically treated patients there were nine reruptures (39%). Six of the 23 patients (26%) treated nonsurgically returned to their previous level of activity, while 37 out of 39 surgically treated patients (95%) did so. Surgical treatment, therefore, is often supported because it yields fewer reruptures and a higher certainty of returning to activity. Superior tendon reconstruction and restoration of function is achieved with surgical repair.[7]

Surgery is to be followed by immobilization, consisting of one month in a long-leg cast with the foot in an equinus position, one month in a short-leg cast with the foot in an equinus position, and then six months using a heel lift.[23]

Problem: Decreased Motion

Range of motion in the ankle and calf decreases following a period of immobilization. Exercises are required to restore motion.

REHABILITATION: RANGE OF MOTION/STRETCHING

In the study by Lea and Smith[14] of the effect of conservative treatment on Achilles tendon ruptures, measurements for the increase in ankle range of motion, specifically dorsiflexion, were taken as indicators for success. Nineteen of 45 patients had symmetrical range of motion.[14]

In 1981, Nistor[19] compared the effects of surgical and conservative treatment on Achilles tendon injuries. Comparisons were made between the range of motion in the injured and uninjured legs. Twenty-seven of 41 surgically treated patients and 40 of 54 patients in the conservatively treated group showed changes of five degrees or less. In each group, 14 patients demonstrated changes in range of motion of 10 degrees or more. The surgically treated patients tended to lose more plantar flexion, while those treated conservatively lost less plantar flexion but gained dorsiflexion. Limitations in the range of motion, as in the results of Lea and Smith,[14] were evident during the toe raises and walking.

Smart et al.[26] recommend plantar and dorsiflexion exercises, circumscribing small circles with the foot, picking up small objects with the toes, and, eventually, performing wall leans.

Range of motion can be accomplished through the calf-stretching exercises described earlier in the section on shin splints. For each exercise the stretched position should be held for 10 seconds, and each exercise should be repeated 15 times, two to three times a day (see Figs 2–11,A-D)

Problem: Decreased Strength and Agility

The ability to bear weight in the toe walking position was used an an indicator for loss of or return to normal strength following treatment for an Achilles tendon rupture. In Lea and Smith's study,[15] subjects demonstrated toe walking 24 weeks after conservative treatment was started. In their 1972 study,[14] 48 of 52 patients were able to bear weight fully on the ball of the foot. All patients were able to bear weight in the study of Lildholdt and Munch-Jorgensen.[17] Both those patients treated conservatively and those treated surgically could demonstrate toe walking in Nistor's 1981 study.[19]

While patients were able to return to full weight-bearing in the above studies, assessment of strength with the Cybex II dynamometer have been used in several studies, both to demonstrate strength loss through treatment, and to compare the loss suffered from conservative treatment to that suffered from operative treatment.

In the 1978 study of Jacobs et al.,[10] which compared the effects of operative treatment to those of conservative treatment, calf strength was assessed by measuring the maximum force in a static condition using a calibrated load cell. The results showed that the operatively treated group demonstrated a better recovery of affected muscle tendon unit than the group treated conservatively. An average of 75% for plantar flexion force was calculated for the operative group, as compared to 65% for the nonoperative group.[10] In his 1981 study, Nistor[19] reported no significant difference between the group treated operatively and that treated conservatively on isokinetic and isometric measurements on the Cybex II.

Based on the results obtained in a comparative study of 48 surgically treated Achilles tendon ruptures, and 31 conservatively treated ruptures, Inglis et al.[7] concluded that surgically treated patients fared better on measurements of strength, power, and endurance than their nonsurgically treated counterparts, and were also more satisfied with their results.

REHABILITATION: STRENGTHENING EXERCISES

Shields et al.[24] report on the results of Cybex strength and power evaluations performed 6 months, 9 months, and 1 year after surgical treatment of Achilles tendon ruptures. At six months postsurgery, there was an average loss of plantar flexion strength of 32%, and a 39% loss of plantar flexion power. The average loss of dorsiflexion strength at six months was 5% and of dorsiflexion power, 19%. It was found that a period of one year was required to regain normal strength. Return to normal activity was possible for 27 of 33 patients. Strength and power deficits were less for those who received treatment earlier. The presence of strength and power deficits, as illustrated in the study above, demonstrates that rehabilitation exercises are necessary. Smart et al.[26] advocate strengthening exercises, including toe raises, and plantar and dorsiflexion exercises on either a Cybex II isokinetic unit or on a leg press machine.

Toe Walking/Raises, Heel Walking/Raises

The instructions for heel and toe walking are included in the section on strengthening that follows the section on stress reaction and stress fractures (see Figs 3–22,A and B and 3–23,A and B).

"Theraband"

For the instructions for the inversion and eversion exercises using the "Theraband," refer to the section on stress fractures and stress reactions (see Figs 3–24,A and B and 3–25,A and B).

Elgin Exercises

Exercises on the Elgin ankle exerciser can also be performed to improve strength.

To Strengthen the Ankle Plantar Flexors

Position.—Begin with the foot in the fully dorsiflexed position (dorsiflexed at 90 degrees). The thigh should not be internally or externally rotated. The weight is placed on the spool closest to the patient (see Fig 3–27,A).

Action.—The patient should then plantar flex the foot until it reaches the fully contracted plantar flexed position (see Fig 3–27,B). Hold the fully contracted position for 2 seconds. Return to the starting position, and repeat for three sets of 10 to 12 repetitions, one to two times a day.

To Strengthen the Ankle Dorsiflexors

Position.—Begin with the foot in the fully plantar flexed position. The weight is placed on the spool furthest from the patient on the vertical axis.

Action.—The patient should then dorsiflex the foot until it reaches the fully contracted dorsiflexed position (see Fig 3–28). Hold the fully contracted position for two seconds. Return to the starting position, and repeat for three sets of 10 to 12 repetitions, one to two times a day.

To Strengthen the Ankle Invertors

Position.—Begin with the ankle in the fully everted position. Again, the knee and thigh should not turn inward but remain straight ahead. The weight should be placed on the spool on the medial side (see Fig 3–29,A).

Action.—The patient should move the foot through the range of motion until it reaches the fully contracted inverted position (see Fig 3–29,B). Hold the fully contracted position for two seconds. Return to the initial position and repeat the exercise for three sets of 10 to 12 repetitions, one to three times a day.

To Strengthen the Ankle Evertors

Position.—Begin with the ankle in the fully inverted position. The weight should be placed on the spool on the lateral side (see Fig 3–30,A).

Action.—The patient should move the foot through the range of motion until it reaches the fully contracted everted position (see Fig 3–30,B). Return to the initial position and repeat the exercise for three sets of 10 to 12 repetitions, one to two times a day.

Cybex

Isokinetic exercises similar to the ones described above can be performed on the Cybex II (see Figs 3–31 through 3–33). A more detailed discussion of isokinetic exercise can be found in Chapter 1.

Wobbleboard

Exercises on the Unidirectional Wobbleboard.—For each of the exercises described below, the athlete is instructed to rock back and forth in a controlled manner for three minutes in each direction.

When exercising the injured leg, the patient is to stand on that leg only. Use a wall or chair for support.

Exercises for Plantar Flexion and Dorsiflexion.—Follow the steps given below.

1. Place the injured foot of the injured leg on the wobbleboard with the axis running perpendicular to the foot (see Fig 3–39,A).
2. Rock back and forth, touching the front edge of the board to the floor, then touching the back edge to the floor, and so on.

Exercises for Inversion and Eversion.—Follow the steps given below.

1. Place the injured foot on the wobbleboard with the axis running vertical to the foot (see Fig 3–39,B).
2. Rock back and forth in a controlled manner, touching the right edge of the board to the floor, then touching the left edge to the floor, and so on.

Exercises for Supination and Pronation in 45 Degrees External Rotation.–Follow the steps given below.

1. Place the injured foot on the wobbleboard diagonally, as shown in Figure 3–39,C.

2. Rock back and forth, touching first the right edge of the board to the floor, then touching the left edge to the floor, and so on.

Exercises for Supination and Pronation in 45 Degrees of Internal Rotation.—Follow the steps given below.

1. Place the foot on the wobbleboard diagonally, as shown in Figure 3–39,D.
2. See step 2 above.

Exercises Using the Multidirectional Wobbleboard.—Follow the steps given below.

1. Place the injured foot on the multidirectional board (see Fig 3–40,A).
2. Using a wall or chair for support, rotate the ankle clockwise, rolling the edge of the board close to the floor, but not touching it (see Fig 3–40,B).
3. Repeat step 2, rotating the ankle in the opposite direction (see Figs 3–40,A and B).

Adhesive Strapping

The Achilles tendon strapping procedure described in the section on Achilles tendinitis can be applied in the case of ruptures also for support following return to activity. Refer to the section on adhesive strapping in the section on Achilles tendinitis that precedes this section. The method for application is described there (see Figs 4–1 through 4–4).

INJURY: GASTROCNEMIUS STRAIN
Problem: Pain

An acute tearing sensation, an audible snap, difficulty in walking, swelling, tenderness, and a palpable defect in the muscle belly, are among the symptoms that can characterize tears of the gastrocnemius.[23] The gastrocnemius can often be strained at its medial head near its musculotendinous junction. It is susceptible to tears, since it works across two joints. Such tearing can occur when the ankle is dorsiflexed and the knee is suddenly extended, as in tennis. This injury is characterized by an acute, sharp pain, aching in the calf, increased pain with dorsiflexion, and tenderness in the medial belly of the muscle.[13]

Problem: Swelling

Swelling has also characterized strains to the gastrocnemius. A 20-minute ice application is also used for strains of the gastrocnemius, for the first 48 to 72 hours.[13, 23, 24, 32] Cold accompanied by compression can be administered via the Jobst Cryo/Temp system. The combination of compression and cold is effective for reducing swelling and inflammation, and relieving pain.

The Jobst Cryo/Temp cold and pressure therapy system allows for the application of cold with or without constant pressure. This accomplished via a flow of coolant to an appliance, which encloses the entire extremity (see Fig 3–16). There are a variety of appliances available for use on all extremity injuries.

The temperature can be adjusted to range from room temperature to 34° F. The pressure can be set from between 0 mm Hg and 160 mm Hg, and can be applied constantly or intermittently, from 0 to 180 seconds on, and 0 to 60 seconds off.

The application of the Jobst Cryo/Temp appliance is as follows:

1. The injured leg should be placed into the appliance. Leg appliances range from half-leg to three-quarter-leg and full-leg lengths.

2. The treatment is normally set between 55° and 70° F.

3. The recommended treatment pressure is set between 80 and 120 mm Hg.

4. The treatment is continued for 20 minutes. The pressure is run intermittently with a ratio of 3:1 on-off time.

5. Jobst treatment may be repeated several times per day.

Problem: Decreased Function

Following resolution of the gastrocnemius strain, a significant loss of ankle motion occurs.

REHABILITATION: STRETCHING

Once pain begins to diminish, calf stretching exercises can begin.[13, 32] Kulund recommends 10 minutes of passive stretching with "Theraband" for 10-second intervals, after the calf has been iced for 20 minutes. Standing calf stretches can be done when swelling and soreness have lessened.[13] The calf stretching exercises and the "Theraband" exercises are described in the sections on stress fractures, stress reactions, and Achilles ruptures. Refer to these sections for methods and illustrations.

REHABILITATION: STRENGTHENING

Strengthening exercises should be a part of the rehabilitation program for this injury.[23, 32] Kulund[13] recommends isometric and manual resistance exercises three times a day. These are implemented after icing, stretching, and ultrasound have been applied. Strengthening exercises can include heel and toe walking, "Theraband," Elgin exercises, wobbleboard, and Cybex exercises.

INJURY: PLANTARIS RUPTURE

The plantaris muscle arises from the lateral condyle of the femur, passes beneath the gastrocnemius and soleus muscles, and then attaches to tendo

Achilles or tubercle of the calcaneus on the medial side. Complete rupture of this muscle will be painful and disabling. Repair is not required, though, because the muscle serves little function. After the acute and inflammatory stage, stretching and strengthening exercises, as described above, are recommended.

REFERENCES

1. Andrews JR: Overuse syndromes of the lower extremity. *Clin Sports Med* 1983; 2:137–148.
2. Bonci CM: Adhesive strapping techniques. *Clin Sports Med* 1982; 1:99–116.
3. Clancy WG, Neidhart D, Brand RL: Achilles tendonitis in runners: A report of five cases. *Am J Sports Med* 1976; 4(2):46–57.
4. Clancy WG: Runner's injuries: II. Evaluation and treatment of specific injuries. *Am J Sports Med* 1980; 8(4):287–289.
5. Eggold JF: Orthotic foot control and the overuse syndrome. *Phys Sports Med,* January 1975, pp 75–79.
6. Gillies H, Chalmers J: The management of fresh ruptures of the tendo achillis. *J Bone Joint Surg Am* 1970; 52:337–343.
7. Inglis AE, Scott WN, Sulco TP, et al: Ruptures of the tendo achillis: An objective assessment of surgical and nonsurgical treatment. *J Bone Joint Surg Am* 1976; 58:990–993.
8. Jackson DW: Shinsplints: An update. *Phys Sports Med,* October 1978, pp 52-61.
9. Jackson DW, Bailey D: Shin splints in the young athlete: A nonspecific diagnosis. *Phys Sports Med,* March 1975, pp 45-51.
10. Jacobs D, Martens M, Van Audekercke R, et al: Comparison of conservative and operative treatment of Achilles tendon rupture. *Am J Sports Med* 1978; 6(3):107–111.
11. James SL, Bates BT, Ostering LR: Injuries to runners. *Am J Sports Med* 1978; 6:40–50.
12. Krissoff WB, Ferris WD: Runner's injuries. *Phys Sports Med* 1979; 7(12):53–64.
13. Kulund DN: The leg, ankle and foot, in Kulund DN (ed): *The Injured Athlete.* Philadelphia, JB Lippincott Co, 1982, pp 425–472.
14. Lea RB, Smith L: Nonsurgical treatment of tendo achillis rupture. *J Bone Joint Surg Am* 1972; 54:1398–1407.
15. Lea RB, Smith L: Rupture of the Achilles tendon: Nonsurgical treatment. *Clin Orthop* Sept-Oct 1968, pp 115–118.
16. Leach RE, James S, Wasilewski S: Achilles tendonitis. *Am J Sports Med* 1981; 9(2):93–98.
17. Lildholdt T, Munch-Jørgensen T: Conservative treatment of Achilles tendon rupture: A follow up study of 14 cases. *Acta Orthop Scand* 1976; 47:454–458.
18. Nistor L: Conservative treatment of fresh subcutaneous rupture of the Achilles tendon. *Acta Orthop Scand* 1976; 47:459–462.
19. Nistor L: Surgical and nonsurgical treatment of Achilles tendon rupture. *J Bone Joint Surg Am* 1981; 63:394–399.
20. O'Donaghue DH: Injuries of the leg, in O'Donaghue DH (ed): *Treatment of the Injured Athlete.* Philadelphia, WB Saunders Co, 1984, pp 586–600.
21. Puranen J: The medial tibial syndrome: Exercise ischaemia in the medial fascial compartment of the leg. *J Bone Joint Surg Br* 1974; 56:712–715.
22. Ryan AJ (moderator), Clancy WG, Detmer DE, et al: Leg pain in runners. *Phys Sports Med* 1977; 5(9):42–53.
23. Shields CL: Achilles tendon injuries and disabling conditions. *Phys Sports Med* 1982; 10(12):77–84.
24. Shields CL, Kerlan RK, Jobe FW, et al: The Cybex II evaluation of surgically repaired Achilles tendon ruptures. *Am J Sports Med* 1978; 6:369–372.

25. Skeoch DU: Spontaneous partial subcutaneous ruptures of the tendo Achillis. *Am J Sports Med* 1981; 9(1):20–21.

26. Smart GW, Taunton JE, Clement DB: Achilles tendon disorders in runners: A review. *Med Sci Sports* 1980; 12(4):231–243.

27. Stein SR, Luekens CA: Closed treatment of Achilles tendon ruptures. *Orthop Clin North Am* 1976; 7:241–246.

28. Subotnick SI: The abuses of orthotics in sports medicine. *Phys Sports Med,* July 1975, pp 73–75.

29. Subotnick SI: Orthotic foot control and the overuse syndrome. *Phys Sports Med,* January 1975, pp 75–79.

30. Taunton JE, Clement DB, Webber D: Lower extremity stress fractures in athletes. *Phys Sports Med* 1981; 9(1):77–86.

31. Turco VJ: Injuries to the ankle and foot in athletics. *Orthop Clin North Am* 1977; 8:669–682.

32. Zarins B, Ciullo JV: Acute muscle and tendon injuries in athletes. *Clin Sports Med* 1983; 2(1):167–182.

CHAPTER 5

The Knee

INJURY: CONTUSION

Contusions to the knee area are sustained in a variety of sports, usually from direct blows. Local swelling, tenderness, ecchymosis, and overlying abrasion can result. Cold packs, compression, and the use of protective padding on return to activity are usually sufficient measures: rehabilitation is not usually necessary. While this injury is fairly simple to resolve, care needs to be taken to ensure that the diagnosis is correct.[10]

INJURY: PREPATELLAR BURSITIS

Direct trauma, such as falling on a flexed knee, can result in this common form of bursitis. The bursa is affected by direct trauma because it lies between the skin and the anterior surface of the patella.[10]

Prepatellar bursitis is usually acute but it can become chronic if it is not adequately treated.

The acute phase of prepatellar bursitis is characterized by immediate swelling, tenderness, redness, and pain with extreme flexion. Inflammation and snowball crepitation may also be present. Ice and compression should be applied, and if necessary, the bursa may be aspirated and a culture of synovial fluid obtained. Protective padding is recommended. Acute bursitis can develop into a chronic condition, characterized by persistent swelling, inflammation, and tenderness. Aspiration, injection of a corticoid, application of a pressure dressing, and possible surgical excision are methods of treatment.[10]

INJURY: CHONDROMALACIA

Chondromalacia of the patella can result from trauma or disturbance of patellar function. It can also develop without an identifiable etiological cause, usually overuse. Chondromalacia is a deterioration or wearing down of the articular cartilage of the patella[10] and can present with four degrees of severity. Grade 1 involves softening of the articular surface; grade 2, fissuring; grade 3, erosion of the articular cartilage; and grade 4, a defect that extends down to the subchondral bone. Symptoms include pain when the knee is extended against resistance, as in the knee extension exercises on a Nautilus or Universal gym. Stair climbing, running hills, or even the simple act of sitting for prolonged periods of time with the knee bent can also be painful. Primary malacia can affect both knees and can result either from patella alta or lateral tracking of the patella as the knee is extended against resistance. Chondromalacia is also characterized by pain and retropatellar crepitation with knee extension while the patella is held firmly against the patellar groove.[10] The patellar inhibition test will verify that chondromalacia is present. The patient should lie supine on the examining table with legs extended and relaxed. Using the "V" of the hand between the thumb and the first finger on the superior aspect of the patella, the examiner pushes the patella distally in the trochlear groove. The patient then tightens the quadricep muscle while the physician provides resistance against patellar excursion. Pain-free, smooth movement indicates a normal knee. Pain with movement and palpable crepitation indicates chondromalacia.[5] Swelling, effusion, crepitation, and locking may be present.

Depending on the severity, chondromalacia can be treated conservatively with ice, aspirin, and by ceasing the offending activity.[10]

REHABILITATION

Individuals with mild cases and a positive patellar inhibition test are limited to isometric straight-leg lifts. When the patellar inhibition test becomes negative, usually after six weeks of the isometric program, the short arc-isotonic quadriceps program may be initiated. These exercises will be described in the following section on patellar tendinitits.

INJURY: PATELLAR TENDINITIS (JUMPER'S KNEE)

Jumper's knee is an overuse injury in which microtears occur at the site of the attachment of the infrapatellar tendon in the inferior pole of the patella. In most instances, treatment consists of ice, isometric quadriceps exercise sets, and activity modification. Occasionally, in cases of refracture, surgical debridement of the tendon may be indicated. Rarely, it may be necessary to excise an intertendinous ossicle.

REHABILITATION

The following exercises are recommended for nonoperative treatment of chondromalacia and patellar tendinitis.

Isometric Straight Leg Lifts

For isometric straight leg lifts, follow the steps given below (Figs 5–1,A and B).

1. Lie supine on a flat surface.
2. Slowly contract the thigh muscles and dorsiflex the foot so that the toe points toward the ceiling.
3. Slowly lift the foot 12 in. up from the surface it rests upon.
4. Hold for 6 seconds.
5. Lower slowly.
6. Continue in this manner completing three sets of ten leg raises with a one-minute rest between each set.

When the 30 leg lifts become easy to do, add 2.5 lb to the ankle and exercise with that weight until it becomes easy. Progress with weights in 2.5-lb increments until it is possible to lift one-tenth of total body weight.

These exercises should be done at least once daily and preferably twice a day (every day). Ice the knee for 20 minutes after each exercise session (see Chapters 1 and 12 for further discussion of cryotherapy).

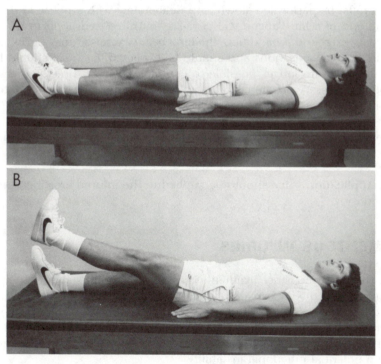

FIG 5–1.
Isometric leg lifts. **A,** the starting position for isometric leg lifts: lay supine on a flat surface, feet and legs together, arms at sides. **B,** contract the quadriceps muscle in the injured leg and lift it 12 in. from the surface it rests on. Hold this position for 6 seconds, lower slowly, rest 6 seconds, then repeat. While performing this exercise, the subject's ankle should be in the neutral position, with the toe toward the ceiling.

Short-Arc Isotonics

Begin in a sitting position with the knee bent about 30 degrees. Slowly extend the leg until it is fully extended. Hold this position for 2 to 4 seconds, slowly lower the leg and relax. Perform a series of three sets of 12 repetitions with the injured leg, alternating with three sets of 12 repetitions with the uninjured leg. Rest 15 minutes, and repeat the entire series.

Starting Weight.—Initially, particularly in injured patients, it is best to start out with the lowest weight possible. If it is easy to do 12 repetitions, add weight. With the correct weight it should be possible to perform 8 to 12 repetitions before fatigue occurs.

Progression.—Ideally, the amount lifted should be increased every seven to ten days. However, this can vary, and is not a hard and fast rule. Progression will be achieved initially by the ability to perform more repetitions before fatigue. Once the maximum number of repetitions listed on the instruction sheet have been reached, increase the weight by 5 to 10 lb.

Fatigue and Lifting Form.—Good lifting form is essential for each repetition and must be performed slowly and deliberately with a pause at the beginning and end of a lift. Fatigue will cause a "burning" sensation in the muscle group being exercised. In addition, the limb being exercised may begin to shake. These are normal sensations and should be expected. Each set should be continued until it is no longer possible to complete at least three-quarters of the full motion necessary on each exercise. It is fairly important to push to the limit and to learn to distinguish between discomfort and pain.

Frequency and Duration.—In the early stages of the program, lifting should be performed twice daily.

Ice Application.—Ice should be applied to the injured area for 20 minutes after exercising.

LIGAMENTOUS INJURIES

Integrity of the various knee ligaments is essential for joint stability. The primary ligaments are the medial capsular, posterior oblique, and the tibial collateral on the medial side; the arcuate and the lateral collateral ligaments on the lateral side; and the anterior cruciate (ACL) and posterior cruciate ligaments (PCL) centrally. Through varying mechanisms these ligaments are subject to injury, resulting in potential functional instability.

A classification[1] of ligamentous injuries based on severity describes them as mild (first-degree), moderate (second-degree) and severe (third-degree). In mild injuries, there is no instability and no increased laxity with stress applied to the knee.[1] Definite tears are present in second-degree injuries, and the injury is characterized by a partial loss of integrity in the ligament complex.[1, 9] Complete tears comprise third-degree sprains and complete integrity of the ligamentous complex is lost.

Problems: Pain, Swelling, Limited Motion

First- and second-degree injuries are associated with pain, swelling, and limited motion. Although effusion may be present, locking and instability are usually absent. First-degree sprains are treated with ice, compression, and rest, with rehabilitation exercises beginning as soon as the patient is relatively comfortable. Depending on degree of joint laxity, second-degree sprains may require immobilization. However, rehabilitation exercises are the essential component of treatment of these injuries. Third-degree injuries generally require surgical repair.

REHABILITATION

Following injury or ligamentous reparative or reconstructive surgery, the following exercise regimens are utilized at the University of Pennsylvania Sports Medicine Center. It is a graduated program to effect range of motion and muscle strength.

Postoperative Program 1

The *postoperative program 1* is initiated in the early post-injury stage in nonsurgical patients and after cast removal in the surgical patient.

Warm-up: Range of Motion.—Follow the steps listed below.

Extension.—Extend the leg until a gentle stretch is felt. Hold this position for 10 seconds. Return the leg to the starting position.

Flexion.—Bend the leg until a gentle stretch is felt. Do not flex the knee beyond 90 degrees. Hold this position for 10 seconds. Return the leg to the starting position.

Alternate between extension and flexion until the completion of 20 repetitions of each exercise.

Leg Lifts.—Follow the steps listed below.

Position 1.—Lie supine on a flat surface. Slowly contract the thigh muscles and dorsiflex the foot so that the toe is pointed back toward the foot. Slowly lift the foot 12 in. Hold it there for 6 seconds, lower slowly (see Figs 5–1,A and B).

Position 2.—Lie on side (opposite the injured knee). Keeping the knee as straight as possible, lift the leg so that the heel is 15 in. above the table surface. Hold the leg in this position for 6 seconds. Then lower the leg and relax (Figs 5–2,A and B).

Repeat this exercise 20 to 25 times. Follow the exercise with 20 minutes of ice application. This program should be done two to three times per day.

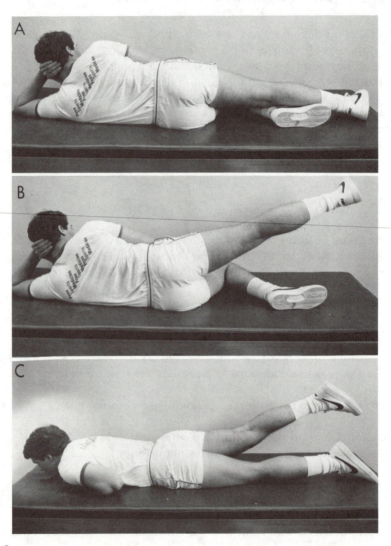

FIG 5–2.
Side leg lifts, position 2. **A,** the starting position for the side leg lift 2. Lie on side with injured leg *(right)* on top. The injured leg is extended and the noninjured leg slightly flexed. **B,** raise the injured leg, keeping the knee as straight as possible, until the heel is 12 in. from the surface. Hold this position for 6 seconds, lower slowly, relax, and repeat. **C,** position 3—lie prone on a flat surface. With the knee in full extension, lift the leg as high as possible (without the hips rolling or lifting off the table). Hold for 6 seconds, relax, and repeat.

Postoperative Program 2

Once range of motion to 90 degrees has been obtained, strengthening can progress from straight-leg raises to bent knee isometrics.

Warm-up: Range of Motion.—Follow the steps listed below.

Extension.—See description in *postoperative program 1*. Repeat 20 times.

Flexion.—See description in *postoperative program 1*. Repeat 20 times.

Leg Extension (Isometrics).—Follow the steps given below.

Position 1.—Sit on a table. Bend the knee to 90 degrees (normal sitting position). Attach a strap around the ankle and to the table leg or cross-band of a table. Try to extend the leg. Apply maximum "pain-free" force for 6 seconds. Repeat this exercise 10 times (Fig 5–3,A).

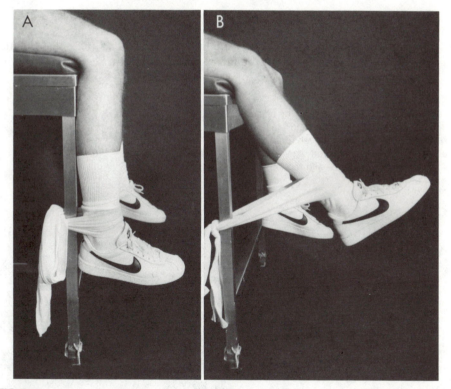

FIG 5–3.
Leg extensions (isometrics). **A,** position 1—sit on the table with the knee flexed to 90 degrees. Attach the leg to the table at the ankle using a strap. Extend the leg against the strap, hold for 6 seconds, relax, and repeat. **B,** position 2—sit on the table with the knee extended to 45 degrees. Again, attach the leg to the table with a strap. Extend the leg against the strap, hold 6 seconds, relax, and repeat.

Position 2.—Sit on a table. Extend the knee 45 degrees. Attach a strap as in position 1. Try to extend the leg. Apply maximum "pain-free" force for 6 seconds. *Do not hold your breath.* Repeat this exercise ten times (Fig 5–3,B). Return to position 1 (90 degrees)—repeat ten times; return to position 2 (45 degrees)—repeat ten times; return to position 1 (90 degrees)—repeat ten times; return to position 2 (45 degrees)—repeat ten times.

Leg Abductions.—In a sitting position, spread the legs apart 12 in. Attach a strap around the thighs just above the knees. Try to spread the legs apart. Squeeze with maximum force for 6 seconds. Do not hold your breath while doing this exercise (Fig 5–4). Repeat this exercise ten times.

Leg Adductions.—In a sitting position, place a ball (basketball, soccer, etc.) between the knees. Squeeze the legs together. Squeeze with maximum force for 6 seconds. Do not hold your breath while doing this exercise (Fig 5–5). Repeat this exercise ten times. Repeat abduction (spread)—ten times; repeat adduction (spread)—ten times.

Leg Lifts.—Follow the steps given below.

Position 1.—Lie supine, and keep the knee as straight as possible. Lift the leg so that the heel is 15 in. above the table surface. Hold the leg in this position

FIG 5–4.
Leg abductions. Sit on a table or chair. Spread the legs 12 in. apart and place a strap around them. Try to spread the legs apart farther, exerting force against the strap for 6 seconds. Relax and repeat.

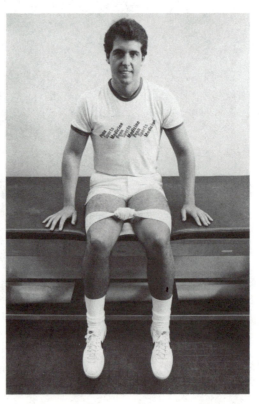

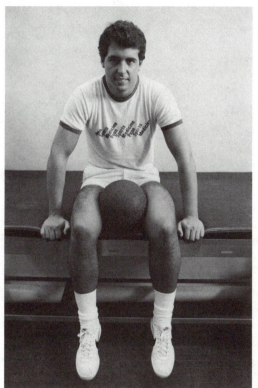

FIG 5–5.
Leg adduction. Sit on a table or chair.
Place a ball between the knees and
squeeze for 6 seconds. Relax and repeat.

for 6 seconds, then lower the leg and relax (see Figs 5–1,A and B). Repeat the exercise 20 to 25 times.

Position 2.—Lie on side (opposite the injured knee). Keep the knee as straight as possible, and lift the leg so that the heel is 15 in. above the table surface. Hold the leg in this position for 6 seconds, then lower the leg and relax (see Figs 5–2,A and B).

Position 3.—Lie prone on stomach, and keep knees as straight as possible. Lift one leg as high as possible, but don't allow the hips to roll or come off the table. Hold this position for 6 seconds. Repeat 15 times (see Fig 5–2,C). Follow this exercise with 20 minutes of ice.

Warm Down: Range of Motion Exercises.—Follow the steps given below.

1. Repeat warm-up procedure (range of motion).
2. Apply ice to the knee—one bag on each side of the knee for 20 minutes.

This program should be done once per day.

Postoperative Program 3

Once the athlete has sufficient range of motion, strength, and ligamentous healing, progressive resistance exercises should be performed as outlined below. These exercises may be done on a Universal gym knee machine, a Nautilus knee extension machine, other knee extension benches, or with a York iron health shoe. This program should follow *postoperative program 2* and may be started when the athlete has good range of motion, minimal pain and swelling, and can bear partial weight.

Nautilus Knee Extension.—Begin in a sitting position, knees aligned with cams (Fig 5–6,A). Slowly extend the leg until it is fully extended (Fig 5–6,B). Hold the leg in the fully extended position for two seconds, then slowly lower it to the starting position.

Leg Lift (Standing).—In a standing position, lift the leg to the front and hold it in this position for 6 seconds; keep the knee straight (Figs 5–7,A and B).

Abduction.—In a sitting position, spread the legs apart 12 in. Attach a strap around the thighs just above the knees. Try to spread the legs apart. Squeeze with maximum force for six seconds. Do not hold your breath while doing this exercise (see Fig 5–4).

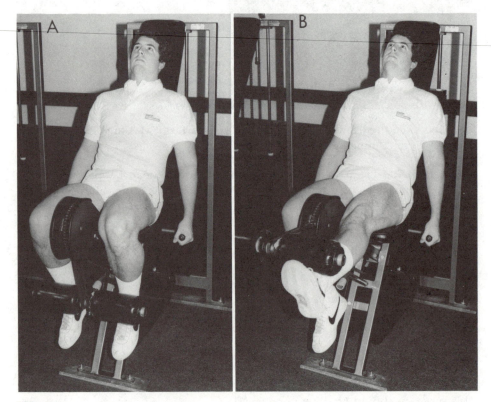

FIG 5–6.
Knee extension—Nautilus. **A,** starting position for knee extension exercises on the Nautilus machine. Flex both knees, align them with the cams, and put the ankles behind the roller. Keep the back and head flat against the machine. **B,** extend the leg through the range of motion to the count of 2, until the leg is in full extension, as shown here. Hold this position for 2 seconds, then lower slowly to the count of 4. Relax and repeat.

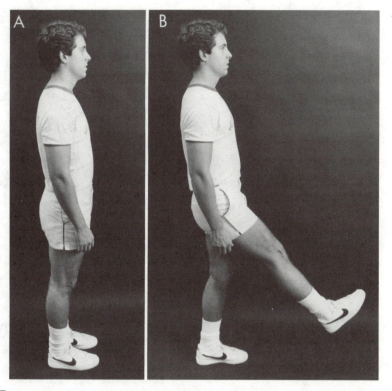

FIG 5–7.
A, the starting position for standing leg lifts. **B,** while standing, lift the leg, keeping it extended, until the foot is off the ground as shown. Hold for 6 seconds, relax, and repeat.

Adduction.—In a sitting position, place a ball (basketball, soccer, etc.) between the knees. Squeeze the legs together. Squeeze with maximum force for 6 seconds. Do not hold your breath while doing this exercise (see Fig 5–5).

Hip Flexion (Standing).—In a standing position, lift the leg up and bend the knee, as if stepping on a stool. Hold it in this position for six seconds (Fig 5–8).

Instructions
Starting Weight.—Initially, particularly in the injured patients, it is best to start out with the lowest weight possible. If it is easy to do 12 repetitions, weight should be added. The correct weight should allow for the performance of eight to ten repetitions before fatigue occurs.

Progression.—Ideally, the amount lifted should increase every seven to ten days. However, this can vary, and it is not a hard and fast rule. Progression will be achieved initially by the ability to perform more repetitions before fatigue. Once the maximum number of repetitions listed on the instruction sheet can be performed, increase the weight by 5 to 10 lb.

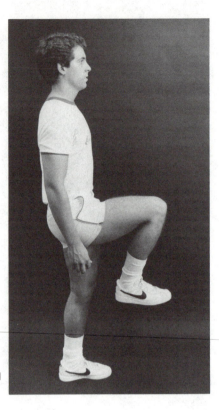

FIG 5–8.
Hip flexion—standing. While standing, lift the leg and bend it at the knee (as if stepping up on a stool). Hold this position for 6 seconds, relax, and repeat.

Fatigue and Lifting Form.—Good lifting is essential for each repetition and must be performed slowly and deliberately with a pause at the beginning and at the end of the lift. Fatigue will cause a "burning" sensation in the muscle group being exercised. In addition, the limb(s) being exercised may begin to shake. These are normal sensations and should be expected. Each set should continue until it is no longer possible to complete at least three-quarters of the full motion necessary on each exercise. It is fairly important to push to the limit, and to learn to distinguish between discomfort and pain.

Frequency and Duration.—In the early stages of the program, lifting should be performed once daily.

Range of Motion Exercises.—These are to be done three to four times a day.

Active assisted range of motion.—Follow the instructions given below.

Extension.—Try to straighten the knee. Extend it to the point at which a "stretch" is felt. Try to extend it further by pushing with the opposite leg. There may be pain. Hold the "stretch" for 10 seconds. Repeat each of these exercises 15 to 20 times (Fig 5–9,A).

Flexion.—Try to bend the knee. Bend it to the point at which a "stretch" is felt. Try to bend it further by pulling with the opposite leg. There may be pain.

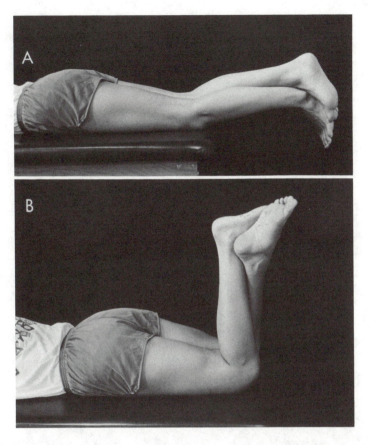

FIG 5–9.
Range of motion. **A,** extension. Try to straighten the knee. Extend it to the point at which a "stretch" is felt. Try to extend it further by pushing with the opposite leg. There may be pain. Hold the "stretch" for 10 seconds. Repeat each of these exercises 15 to 20 times. **B,** flexion. Try to bend the knee. Bend it to the point at which a "stretch" is felt. Try to bend it further by pulling with the opposite leg. There may be pain. Hold the "stretch" for 10 seconds. Repeat each exercise 15 to 20 times.

Hold the stretch for 10 seconds. Repeat each exercise 15 to 20 times (Fig 5–9,B).

Forceful passive range of motion.—If additional assistance is needed, it can be provided by an athletic trainer or physical therapist. A slow, forceful push should be held for 10 to 15 seconds. This method is used in difficult cases of knee flexion contractures following surgery. Forceful passive range of motion should be used in the later stages of rehabilitation when further increases in range of motion are not possible through active or assisted methods (Figs 5–10, A and B).

The program outlined below should be done once every day:

1. Range of motion—15 to 20 repetitions
2. Knee extension (quadriceps)
   Injured leg—12 repetitions
   Uninjured leg—12 repetitions

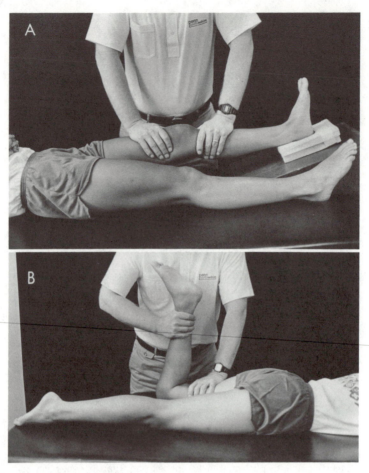

FIG 5–10.
Forceful passive range of motion. **A,** forceful passive range of motion for increasing knee extension.
B, forceful passive range of motion for increasing knee flexion.

    Repeat this sequence two more times
  3. Leg lifts (standing)
    Front—15 to 20 repetitions
    Side—15 to 20 repetitions
    Back—15 to 20 repetitions
  4. Abduction (belt)
    Twelve repetitions
  5. Adduction (ball)
    Twelve repetitions
  6. Knee extension
    Repeat item 2 above
  7. Hip flexion (standing)
    Fifteen to 20 repetitions
  8. Toe raises
    Twenty to 25 repetitions

9. Range of motion (as in the warm-up)
   Fifteen to 20 repetitions for flexion and extension

Following this exercise program, ice should be applied to both sides of the knee for 20 minutes.

The program outlined below may be substituted for *postoperative program 2* or may be used as a general strengthening/conditioning program for the knee and thigh.

Postoperative Program 4: General Strengthening/Conditioning Program

1. Knee extension (quadriceps) (on machine—see description in postoperative program 3)
   Uninjured leg—12 repetitions
   Injured leg—12 repetitions
   Repeat this sequence two more times
2. Knee flexion (hamstrings)
   When using a machine, begin in the prone position, knees aligned with cams. Slowly pull both heels toward the buttocks. Hold for 2 seconds, then slowly return to a starting position. When using a weight shoe begin in a standing position. Lift leg so that the heel touches buttocks. Hold for 2 seconds, then slowly lower (Figs 5–11,A and B).
3. Abduction (belt)
   Twelve repetitions
4. Adduction (ball)
   Twelve repetitions
5. Knee extension
   Repeat step 1 above
6. Knee flexion
   Repeat step 2 above
7. Abduction (belt)
   Repeat step 3 above
8. Adduction (ball)
   Repeat step 4 above

Ice should be applied to the injured area for 20 minutes after exercising.

As with *postoperative program 3*, this program consists of knee extension and flexion, and hip adduction and abduction exercises. Refer to *postoperative program 3* for descriptions of the positions and methods. In addition to the instructions provided in that section, the following comments are important.

Lift as much weight as possible every work out. The first two to three sets may be easy and it may be possible to complete all 12 repetitions. However, the remaining sets should be more difficult and it may not be possible to complete all 12 repetitions in each set. A set should be continued if it is possible to extend the knee at least three-quarters of the way to full extension. If it is possible to complete all 12 repetitions in all six sets, not enough weight is being used. If this is the case, add 5 to 10 lb. When it is possible to complete all 12 repetitions in all six sets with this additional weight, add another 5 to 10 lb. Continue to progress in this manner.

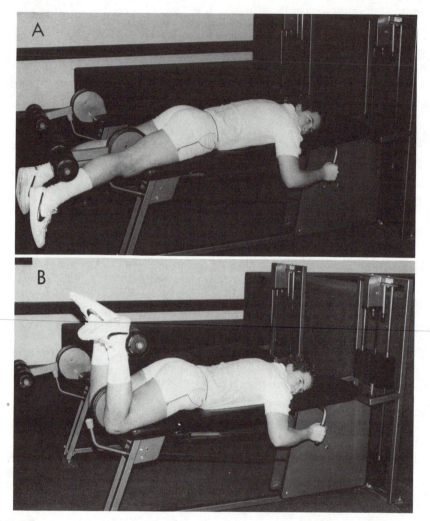

FIG 5–11.
Knee flexion. **A,** starting position for knee flexion exercises using the Nautilus machine. Lie on your stomach. Place both legs under the rollers, and align the joint line with the cam of the machine. Hold on to the handle for support only, and rest the head as shown. **B,** flex the knees and pull the heels toward the buttocks to the count of 2. Hold the flexed position for 2 seconds, and lower slowly to the count of 4. Relax and repeat.

To increase the strength and size of the leg, the muscles must be worked to fatigue within the prescribed number of repetitions (12). If the leg is worked to fatigue there will be a burning sensation in the muscles and they may begin to shake. The legs should feel weak after the workout is over. If these sensations do not occur, workout intensity should be increased. If this is the case, add more weight as outlined above.

Eventually the individual will be able to participate in various forms of activity. Among our recommendations are swimming, cycling, and agility exercises. The role of cycling for knee rehabilitation is discussed by McLeod and Blackburn.[8]

Postoperative Program 5: Agility Program

Warm-up.—Do a quarter to a half mile of easy jogging (8 to 10 min/mile).

Agility.—Perform the following steps:

1. Three to five 10-yd sprints at half speed.
2. Three to five 10-yd sprints at three-quarter speed.
3. Three to five 40-yd sprints at three-quarter speed.
4. Five circles to the right (start with a 10-yd diameter) (see Fig 3–34).
5. Five circles to the left (decrease to a 5-yd diameter circle) (see Fig 3–34).
6. Five to ten figure-of-eights (5-yd diameter circles) (see Fig 3–35).
7. Five boxes to the right (5-yd squares) (see Fig 3–36).
8. Five boxes to the left (5-yd squares) (see Fig 3–36).
9. Five- to 10-yd backward sprints at half speed.
10. Three to five cariocas to the right (20 yd at half speed) (see Fig 3–37).
11. Three to five cariocas to the left (20 yd at half speed) (see Fig 3–37).
12. One 100-yd sprint at half speed.
13. One 100-yd sprint at three-quarter speed.

Warm-Down.—Do a quarter to a half mile of easy jogging (8 to 10 min/ mile).

Try to increase the intensity of the drills as the legs permit. Don't overdo it! If there is pain during the workout, stop and apply ice to the knees for 20 minutes. Resume activity the following day. The program should be followed: daily/three times weekly/other (see Figs 3–34 through 3–37).

Agility programs can also include activities in the water. These can include: (1) flutter kick, (2) bicycle leg motion, (3) running in waist-deep water, (4) lateral shuffle and crossover, and (5) high stepping. Individuals with (1) 15 degrees of extension and 90 degrees of flexion, (2) about 50% of normal extremity strength, (3) a properly fitting brace and (4) motivation can begin this phase of rehabilitation.[2]

THIRD-DEGREE SPRAINS

As with various other athletic injuries there is often controversy as to whether treatment for severe sprains should be conservative or surgical. In either case, it is apparent from the various literature reviews that movement is favorable. Among the authors who provide discussions on nonoperative rehabilitation are Steadman,[14, 15] Hastings,[4] and Indelicato.[6] Yocum et al.,[16] Steadman,[14, 15] Savastano,[12] and Campbell and Glenn[2] provide discussions on postoperative rehabilitation.

REHABILITATION

Regardless of the treatment, rehabilitation principles remain constant. The only variable is the length of immobilization. The same rehabilitation program outlined for grade 1 and 2 injuries should be followed: (1) *postoperative program 1*; (2) *postoperative program 2*; (3) *postoperative program 3*; (4) *postoperative program 4*; and (5) *postoperative program 5* (agility).

In surgical cases involving knee arthrotomy, postoperative recovery may be slow even in the athlete who is motivated to return to athletic competition as rapidly as possible. Athletic participation is not permitted until the range of motion is normal and the strength of the leg that has been operated on is equal to that of the other leg. In some cases, recovery may be influenced by litigation, duration of symptoms prior to surgery, age of the patient, nature of athletic competition, and postoperative complications.[12]

With regard to rehabilitation following anterior cruciate ligament (ACL) repair and/or reconstruction, it should be noted that many orthopedic surgeons do not prescribe the quadriceps exercises described in this book. The trainer/ therapist should consult with the physician concerning this matter.

Some surgeons will treat knee instability with bracing. The C.Ti. and Lenox Hill braces are discussed at the end of this chapter.

MENISCAL INJURIES

In addition to injuries to the bones, tendons, and ligaments, there more commonly occurs damage to the menisci. The function of the medial and lateral menisci include stabilizing the joint, shock absorption, nutrition, and weight bearing. Significant load-transmitting forces are carried by the menisci and range from 40% to 60% of the weight superimposed across the joint.

Rotation of the flexed knee as it moves toward extension can result in traumatic lesions of one or both menisci. This can result in pain along the medial or lateral joint line, effusion, locking, and positive responses to both the Mc-Murray and Ashly tests.[9]

Tears of the medial and/or lateral menisci can occur as isolated phenomenon or in association with ligamentous injuries. Most commonly, ACL tears are associated with meniscal derangement.

Once the meniscal tear has been diagnosed, there are several options for treatment. The physician may elect to simply observe the athlete. This is the least likely course of action to be taken. The physician may elect to repair the torn cartilage if the injury occurs in the peripheral section (outer border) of the meniscus. The physician may elect to completely remove the meniscus or remove only the torn segment. Resection of the meniscus, either partial or total, can, in most instances, be performed through the arthroscope.

With the advent of arthroscopic surgery, surgical management has resulted in marked acceleration of the rehabilitation course.

Isolated injury to either menisci are most effectively treated by surgical arthroscopic technique. Seven to ten days after partial arthroscopic meniscectomy the patient is placed on *postoperative program 2* exercises as described previously. Patients follow the postoperative procedure as outlined for ligamentous injuries. Recovery from meniscal injuries is usually more rapid than from ligamentous injuries.

POSTOPERATIVE TREATMENT AND REHABILITATION

Follow the rehabilitation programs outlined under ligamentous injuries: (1) *postoperative program 2*; (2) *postoperative program 3*; and (3) *postoperative program 5 (agility)*.

FRACTURES

Among the fractures that commonly occur in the knee area are condylar and osteochondral, patellar, and epiphyseal, and fabella fractures.

Chondral fractures are somewhat difficult to diagnose. This injury involves the articular cartilage and can be confused with meniscal tears or osteochondritis dessicans. The femoral chondyles are second to the patella in susceptibility to injury.

The symptoms characterizing these injuries are pain in flexion and extension due to the tense hemarthrosis. Inability to extend the knee represents disruption of the quadriceps mechanism.

Patellar fractures can result from several different mechanisms, including direct-blow injuries, patellar subluxations or dislocations, and chronic stress.

Avulsion fractures of the anterior tibial spines can involve the insertion of the ACL. Open reduction will be necessary if the spine is completely avulsed.

Surgical reduction and fixation may be necessary for a displaced patella.

REHABILITATION

Rehabilitation should include: (1) isometric straight leg raises, (2) *postoperative programs 1* and *2*, (3) *postoperative program 3*, and (4) *postoperative program 5* (agility). Refer to the description of these exercises earlier in this chapter.

INJURY: HAMSTRING STRAINS

The hamstring muscles, located at the posterior aspect of the thigh, produce extension of the hip and flexion of the knee. This muscle group is made up of three separate muscles: (1) semimembranosus, (2) semitendinosus, and (3) biceps femoris.

The origin of this group of muscles is the ischium, the most distal part of the pelvis. The muscles insert behind the knee. The semimembranosus and semitendinosus insert on the medial aspect of the tibia, while the biceps femoris inserts on the lateral aspect of the fibula.

Injuries to this muscle complex are usually due to traction. The mechanism of injury usually affects the muscle belly itself or the origin of the muscle. Rarely does it affect the muscle insertion. On occasion an athlete may fracture the origin of the muscle off the ischium in what is called an avulsion fracture. These injuries commonly occur in sprinters, gymnasts, basketball players, and other athletes who extend their hips. In runners, a long stride or a sudden start place a great deal of stress on the hamstring muscle, and this may cause injury.

Problem: Tenderness, Swelling

When the muscle is injured, there is tenderness associated with a large area of swelling and ecchymosis. On palpation, a defect in the muscle may be noticed. To test the muscle, place the athlete face down on the table and apply gentle resistance against knee flexion and hip extension. The athlete will experience some discomfort. In addition, compare the strength of the injured leg to that of the uninjured leg.

Initially treatment consists of ice and rest. Further athletic activity may increase damage to the muscle, and heat should never be applied. Further athletic activity may not be allowed if the athlete has pain with flexion of the knee or extension of the hip against resistance.

REHABILITATION

Once the acute injury has resolved, hamstring stretches are the hallmark of further treatment. The athlete must stretch diligently before participating and ice the area after activities. Hamstring stretches must be followed by strengthening exercises. Certain athletes are predisposed to recurrent hamstring injuries, and they must stretch prior to all sports, keeping as limber as possible.

When an avulsion fracture occurs, the initial treatment is the same followed by stretching exercises. In a small percentage of cases the bone will not heal by itself, and this may be painful. In this case, surgery may be necessary to relieve the pain. As stated above, most hamstring injuries are treated by nonsurgical means, and prevention is the key to stopping reinjury.

Stretching

There are a number of different stretching techniques for the hamstrings. Several exercises stretch both the hamstrings and groin area (both descriptions and illustrations can be found in Chapter 6). The stretching exercises described below are specifically for the hamstrings.

Hamstring and Calf Stretch

In a standing position, keep both legs straight, feet apart slightly. Bend over at the waist and try to touch the palms of the hands to the floor (Figs 5–12,A and B). Hold this stretch for 10 seconds. Relax and repeat five to ten times.

Hamstring and Calf Stretch—Variation

A variation on this stretch is to cross one leg over the other and bend over to touch the floor. There should be a stretch in the back leg, which should be kept straight (see Figs 5–13,A and B). If it is not possible to touch the floor, reach

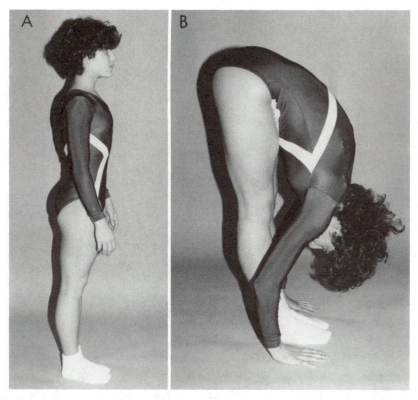

FIG 5–12.
A, starting position for the standing hamstring stretch. **B,** standing hamstring stretch. Keeping the legs straight, bend forward at the waist, and reach toward the floor until there is a stretch in the back of the thighs and behind the knees. Attempt to touch the floor or grasp the ankles. If it is not possible to reach this far without bending the legs, then reach for the midcalf. Hold the stretch for 10 seconds, return to the starting position, then repeat.

down as far as possible until there is a stretch. Hold as above, relax, and repeat. Continue to stretch and try to shorten the distance to the floor.

Hamstring Stretch

In a standing position, place one leg on an object that is higher than the waist. Keep both legs straight. Lean forward until a stretch is felt. Try to grasp the ankle of the elevated leg and attempt to touch the chest and nose to the knee. Switch leg positions with opposite leg. Hold each stretch for 10 seconds. Repeat this exercise five to ten times.

Hurdler's Stretch–Hamstring

Sit in a hurdler's position, with one leg extended forward and the other leg bent so that the sole of the foot touches the inside of the opposite leg. Sit on the buttocks (Fig 5–14,A). Lean forward until a stretch is felt and attempt to grasp the ankle (Fig 5–14,B) or touch the nose to the knee (Fig 5–14,C).

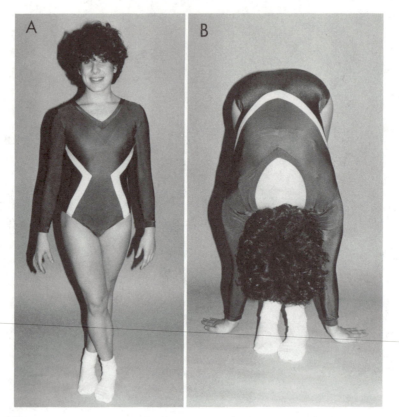

FIG 5–13.
A, starting position for the standing hamstring stretch variation. **B,** with the right leg crossed over the left at the ankle, bend forward at the waist and reach down toward the floor until there is a stretch behind the knees. Attempt to touch the floor or grasp the ankles. If it is not possible to reach down this far, grasp the leg at midcalf. While the front leg may bend slightly, the back leg should remain straight. Hold the stretch for 10 seconds. Return to start and repeat.

Strengthening Exercises

In addition to stretching, strengthening the hamstrings is important. Refer to the postoperative *program 2* and the isotonic knee program for descriptions and illustrations of knee flexion exercises. For warming up, a series of ten stretches for 6 to 10 seconds each is suggested. Stretching is important after working out as well as before.

QUADRICEPS INJURIES

QUADRICEPS CONTUSIONS

Direct impact by an external force, such as a helmet or a knee, to the thigh, can result in a quadriceps contusion. This is a frequent occurrence in football and soccer. The trauma causes bleeding and the formation of a pool of blood known

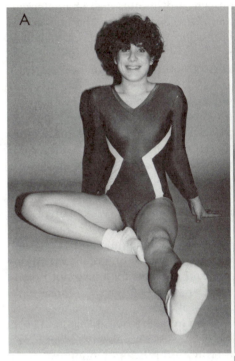
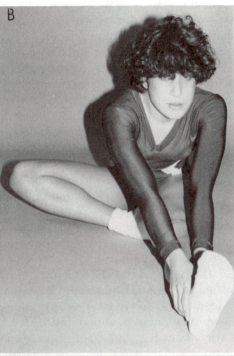
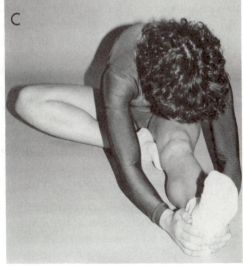

FIG 5–14.
Hamstring hurdler's stretch. **A,** starting
position. Sit on the floor, extend the right leg
in front, and bend the left leg so that the
sole of the shoe touches the inside of the
right leg. **B,** bend forward from the waist,
reaching over the right leg toward the foot.
Reach until there is a stretch behind the
knee. Try to grab the ankle or midcalf. Keep
the right leg straight. Hold the stretched
position for 10 seconds. Relax and repeat.
C, the hurdler's stretch with the chest and
chin to the knee.

as a hematoma. Such injuries can be quite debilitating, and have the potential
of developing into the more serious condition known as myositis ossificans.
Myositis ossificans involves heterotopic bone formation, which is usually visible
on roentgenogram two to four weeks postinjury.

Quadriceps contusions can be classified as mild, moderate, or severe.[7] A
mild injury has been sustained if there is local tenderness, knee motion greater
than 90 degrees, and a normal walking gait. Limitation of knee motion to less

than 90 degrees indicates a moderate contusion; this level is also characterized by a swollen, tender muscle mass and an antalgic gait. Motion is limited to less than 45 degrees in the cases of severe contusions, and the patient will have tenderness and swelling and a severe limp.[7]

Jackson and Feagin[7] report on 65 cases of contusions sustained by West Point cadets between September 1969 and June 1970. Forty-seven patients had mild injuries, and were disabled anywhere from two to 25 days (average, 6.5 days). Disability for seven cadets with moderate injuries ranged from 33 to 95 days (average, 56 days). Eleven cadets had severe injuries, and disability averaged 72 days, with a range from 28 to 180 days. Of the 18 cadets with severe and moderate injuries, ten were hospitalized. Hospitalization was an alternative to bed rest, which was not possible in the barracks. Six of these ten developed myositis ossificans, as did seven of the eight not immobilized. Jackson and Feagin describe three types of myositis ossificans: (1) a type in which there is a stalked connection to the adjacent femur; (2) periosteal type, with total continuity between the heterotopic bone and the adjacent femur; and (3) broad-based type with a portion of ectopic bone projecting into the quadriceps muscle. Disability was 55 days for those hospitalized, 80 days for those not hospitalized, 73 days for those with myositis ossificans, and 49 days for those with moderate and severe injuries but no myositis ossificans.

A three-phase treatment protocol is provided by Jackson and Feagin.[7] Phase 1 consists of ICE and quadriceps isometric exercises. The aim is to minimize hemorrhage; therefore, massage, heat, diathermy, and range-of-motion exercises are contraindicated. Ice and rest are indicated in the acute phase, whereas ice and exercise are indicated later. In the acute phase, we prescribe dexamethasone (Decadron), 0.75 mg, two tablets four times daily for three days. In the study by Jackson and Feagin of 65 cadets, phase 1 lasted 24 hours for mild contusions and 48 hours for moderate injuries. Progression to phase 2 can be made when the condition is stabilized and quadriceps control has been regained. The purpose of this phase is to restore range of motion; emphasis is placed on restoring extension, with flexion exercises included as well. When motion beyond 90 degrees is possible, phase 2 is complete and progression can be made to phase 3, which is the functional rehabilitation phase involving progressive rehabilitation exercises.

Four principles[7] for successful treatment are:

1. It is important to recognize and classify the severity of the initial injury early, and to restrict activity accordingly.
2. Patients with moderate and severe injuries should be restricted to bed rest, ice and elevation, or hospitalization, for at least 48 hours.
3. Precautions should be taken to avoid reinjury during the recovery phase.
4. Regaining full knee extension and quadriceps strength should be emphasized. Caution should be taken in implementing knee flexion exercises; performing knee flexion too soon and too aggressively can cause reinjury.

Myositis ossificans is a serious injury and demands observation and treatment by a physician. Proper care of a thigh contusion will prevent the formation of myositis ossificans. Ice should be used because heat will cause progression of the bleeding process. If the athlete limps, have him use crutches.

Do not massage or stretch the muscle during the acute phase. These two techniques can cause more damage and increase the athlete's "down time."

It is important to stretch the quadriceps muscle group, as described following the discussion of quadriceps strains once the ossification has become quiescent, as evident by the absence of warmth and tenderness.

The athlete may return to competition if he has full range of motion, near-equal strength, is wearing a protective pad, and can meet the demands of the particular sport.[4]

QUADRICEPS STRAINS

As with other muscle groups in the body, the quadriceps is susceptible to strain. Failure to warm up properly and to stretch can result in an injury that otherwise might have been avoided. When excessive demands are placed on the quadriceps, strain can result.

Treatment should consist of ice application and rest. After 48 hours heat can be applied prior to activity. Support can be provided during the initial return to activity through the use of elastic bandaging. In addition to providing support, it also serves as a physical reminder to the athlete that the injury is not completely healed, and to avoid premature overexertion. Flexibility can be improved through stretching the quadriceps.

REHABILITATION

Stretching.—The following exercise will stretch the quadriceps muscle group and can be used both for daily warm-ups of the noninjured athlete, and stretching for quadriceps contusions and strains.

Quadriceps stretch.—In a standing position, flex one leg, bring it up behind, and grasp the ankle. Pull the heel as close to the buttocks as possible until a "stretch" is felt in the thigh. Hold this position for 10 seconds. Relax and repeat these exercises five to ten times (Fig 5–15).

Quadriceps stretch—variation.—A second stretch can be done from a kneeling position on the floor. Begin kneeling with buttocks on the heels (Fig 5–16,A). Lean backward, using the arms for support, creating a straight line from the torso to the knees (Fig 5–16,B). There should be a stretch in the front of the thighs. If it is possible to stretch farther, lean back until resting on elbows (Fig 5–16,C).

Strengthening Exercises.—A weakened quadricep can be strengthened through either isometric quadriceps exercises, or isotonic exercises. Refer to the description and illustration included in postoperative *program 3*.

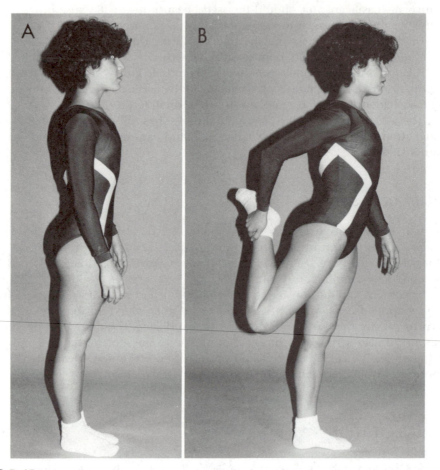

FIG 5–15.
A, starting position for the quadriceps stretch. **B,** while standing, flex the knee and grasp the ankle with the hand. Gently extend the hip until a stretch is felt in the quadriceps muscle. Hold for 10 seconds. Relax and repeat.

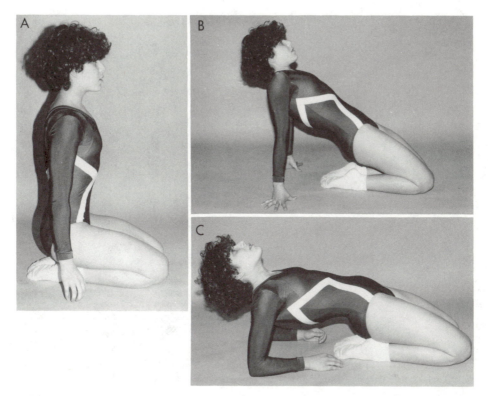

FIG 5–16.
A, starting position for the quadriceps stretch variation. Begin kneeling, legs together. Rest buttocks on heels. **B,** quadriceps stretch variation. From the starting position in **A,** lean backward, using the arms for support, keeping the torso in a straight line with the thighs. There should be a stretch in the front of the thighs. Hold the stretch for 10 seconds. Relax and repeat. **C,** quadricep stretch variation continued. If possible, continue to lean farther backward, and rest on the elbows. Again, a stretch should be felt in the front of the thighs. Hold the stretch for 10 seconds. Relax and repeat.

BRACING

THE C.Ti. BRACE

*Indications**

The C.Ti. brace (Fig 5–17) has been designed to protect for medial, lateral, anterior, posterior, and combined ligament instabilities. Its unique static support system also provides excellent rotary stability. The utilization of a rigid frame and nonelastic straps keeps the knee from hyperextending or deflecting beyond normal range. Medial and lateral support is optimized through a six-point system. The combination of the graphite frame and its lateral arms, condylar support at each side of the joint, and the nonelastic straps simultaneously work to inhibit medial and lateral instability. Anterior-posterior excursion of the tibia is controlled by the graphite tibial member in conjunction with the nonelastic straps. Rotary support is achieved through a combination of the shape

*Reprinted from manufacturer's instructions (Innovation Sports, Irvine, Calif.), with permission.

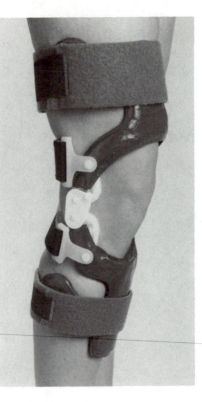

FIG 5–17.
Lateral view of the C.Ti. brace.

of the rigid graphite frame, the nonelastic straps, and the pneumatic and condylar pads at the joint. Pivotal movement of the joint is prevented by the frame, which is fabricated with the tibial member encompassing the tibial crest, the high-strength upright support on each side of the joint, and the femoral member with its lateral arm. The pneumatic and condylar pads provide close support at the joint line.

MEASURING INSTRUCTION FOR THE C.Ti. BRACE

M-L Tracing

1. Place the tracing chart on a hard, flat surface—either an unpadded examining table or the Innovation Sports tracing board. Position the patient's leg with the back of the knee approximately over the fold in the chart. The leg must be fully extended (Fig 5–18,A).
2. Locate and mark the medial joint line on the patient's leg (Fig 5–18,B).
3. To assure that the leg is not internally or externally rotated, flex and extend the patient's leg several times and lower it in a perpendicular line down to the chart (Fig 5–18,C).
4. With the knee in extension, have the patient dorsiflex the foot and contract the quadriceps. This avoids false enlargement of the leg's image due to spread of the flesh. Maintain this contracted position throughout the M-L tracing (Fig 5–18,D).

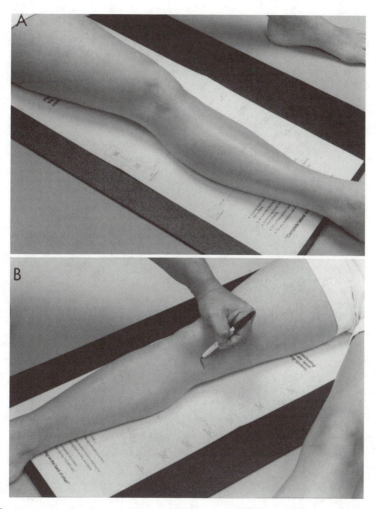

FIG 5–18.
M-L tracing. **A,** the patient's leg is positioned with the back of the knee approximately over the fold in the chart. The leg must be fully extended. **B,** the medial joint line on the patient's leg is located and marked. *(Continued.)*

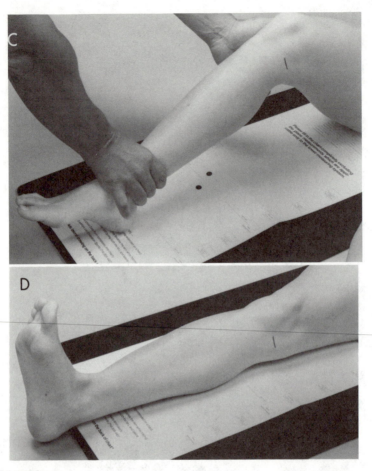

FIG 5–18 (cont.).
C, to ensure that the leg is not internally or externally rotated, the patient's leg is flexed and extended several times and lowered in a perpendicular line down to the chart. **D,** with the knee in extension, the patient should dorsiflex the foot and contract the quadricep to avoid a false enlargement of the leg's image due to spread of the flesh. This contracted position should be maintained throughout the M-L tracing. *(Continued.)*

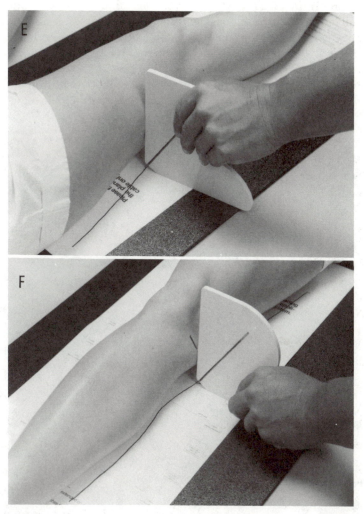

FIG 5–18 (cont.).
E, the tool is positioned at a right angle to the leg with the smaller portion of the handle nearest the chart so that the medial and alteral borders of the leg can be traced. The tool should just barely brush the skin while tracing. **F,** the position corresponding to the medial joint line is marked on the chart.

5. To trace the medial and lateral borders of the leg, position the tool at a right angle to the leg with the smaller portion of the handle nearest the chart. The tool should just barely brush the skin while tracing (Fig 5–18,E).
6. Next, mark the position corresponding to the medial joint line on the chart (Fig 5–18,F).

Tibial Measurements

7. To complete the tibial measurements, mark the tibial crest at points approximately corresponding to the two tibial measurement boxes lo-

cated on the chart (Fig 5–19,A). (The leg should remain in the contracted position for steps A and B.)

8. Set the tracing tool against the lateral side of the leg and along the line
extending from the tibial measurement box. Using a measuring tape,
read the distance from the edge of the tracing tool to the crest of the
tibia. Repeat this procedure for the upper tibial measurement. Record
these numbers in the appropriate locations on the chart (Fig 5–19,B).

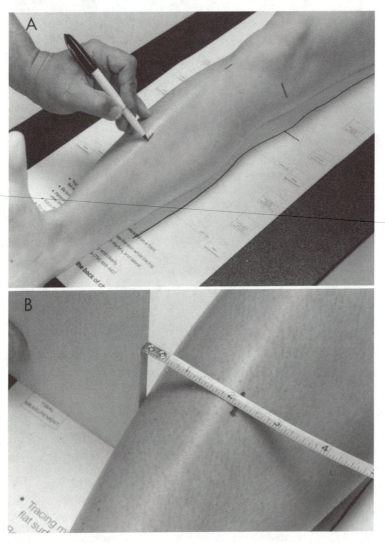

FIG 5–19.
A, the tibial crest is marked at points approximately corresponding to the two tibial measurement
boxes located on the chart. The leg should remain in the contracted position for steps **A** and **B. B,**
the tracing tool is set against the lateral side of the leg and along the line extending from the tibial
measurement box. With a measuring tape, the distance from the edge of the tracing tool to the crest
of the tibia is read. This procedure is repeated for the upper tibial measurement. These numbers
should be recorded in the appropriate locations on the chart.

Circumference Measurements

9. Measure the girth of the knee just below the distal border of the patella (at the popliteal crease and patellar tendon). Record this measurement in the box labeled "distal pole." Next, mark, measure, and record the circumference of the leg at 3 in. and 6 in. above and below midpatella (Fig 5–20).

A-P Tracing

10. Turn the chart over to the unmarked side and place the leg lateral-side down on the chart anywhere in the range between 5 and 20 degrees of flexion (Fig 5–21,A).
11. With the tool, trace the anterior and posterior borders of the leg. Again, be sure that the tool just barely brushes the skin while tracing (Fig 5–21,B).
12. Finally, locate the proximal and distal borders of the patella and mark lines corresponding to these points on the chart (Fig 5–21,C).

Ordering Information

For assistance during the tracing procedure, contact Innovations Sports' customer service (1-800-222-4CTi outside California, and 1-800-331-5491 within California). Customer service is available Monday through Friday from 9 A.M. to 5 P.M., Pacific Standard Time. Further information is available from Innovation Sports, 15801 Rockfield Blvd., Suite E, Irvine, CA 92718.

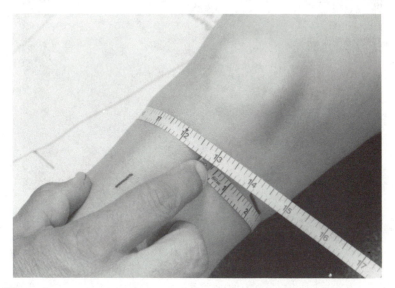

FIG 5–20.
Circumference measurements. The girth of the knee just below the distal border of the patella is measured (at the popliteal crease and patellar tendon). This measurement should be recorded in the box labeled "distal pole." The circumference of the leg, at 3 and 6 in. *above and below* the midpatella is marked, measured, and recorded.

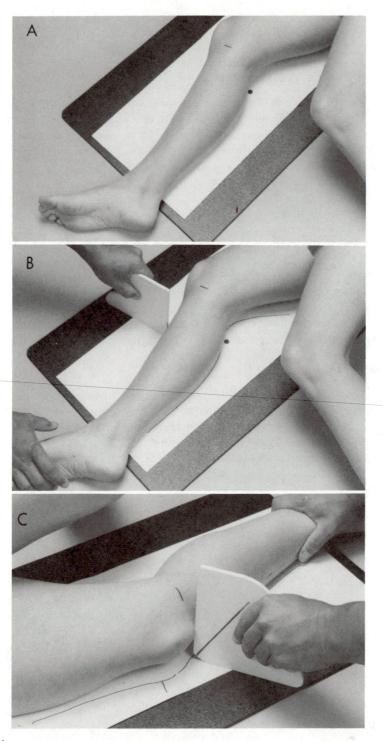

FIG 5–21.
A-P tracing. **A,** the chart is turned over to the unmarked side and the leg is placed lateral side down on the chart anywhere in the range between 5 and 20 degrees of flexion. **B,** with the tool, the anterior and posterior borders of the leg are traced. Again, be sure the tool just barely brushes the skin while tracing. **C,** finally, the proximal and distal borders of the patella are located and lines corresponding to these points are marked on the chart.

LENOX HILL DEROTATION BRACE (PLASTER MODEL)

Indications

The Lenox Hill derotation brace is used to compensate for posttraumatic ligament laxity and instability, as well as to protect the knee from surgery.

Instructions: Plaster Model*

1. Apply a 4-in. cotton stockinette to the extended leg (full extension requested but *not* necessary for casting) (Fig 5–22,A).
2. With a moistened indelible pencil, outline the patella and the fibula head (Fig 5–22,B).
3. Outline the tibia (Fig 5–22,C).
4. Make vertical and transverse lines through the knee center (Fig 5–22,D).
5. Bisect transverse line, lateral and medial (Fig 5–22,E).
6. Mark 8 in. above and 8 in. below the knee center. Cast *must* be at least this length (Fig 5–22,F).
7. Apply a 1 in. cutting strip lateral to the patella (webbing, felt, or your choice) (Fig 5–22,G).
8. Wrap with *plaster* bandage (not synthetic). For the average leg, 2 rolls of 6 in. bandage and one roll of 4 in. bandage (Fig 5–22,H). Write patient's name on the cast.
9. Make a series of horizontal lines over site of the cutting strip (Fig 5–22,I).
10. Univalve the cast (Fig 5–22,J).
11. Remove the cutting strip and cut the stockinette (Fig 5–22,K).
12. Spring the cast off the leg, remove, and discard the stockinette (if indelible pencil was *not* used, leave stockinette in cast) (Fig 5–22,L).
13. Tape closed and cut the cast back to 8 in. marks (refer to Figure 5–23,F) (Fig 5–22,M).
14. Complete the prescription form and staple it and other paperwork inside the cast (Fig 5–22,N). Fill in and around the cast with packing material to protect in shipment.
15. Place in reusable carton from the last brace delivery (Fig 5–22,O).

Application Instructions*

1. Align the axis of the brace with the anatomical axis (Fig 5–23,A). On those few braces prescribed for varus (lateral instability), the long straight bar runs along the inside of the knee.
2. Place the medial derotation strap under the pretibial bar (Fig 5–23,B). (Some braces may be prescribed to have only one derotation brace.)
3. Cross the lateral derotation strap over the medial strap and secure with the distal patella pad (Fig 5–23,C).
4. Secure the proximal patella pad (Fig 5–23,D).
5. The posterior view of patella straps shown parallel (Fig 5–23,E).

---

*From the manufacturer's instructions (Lenox Hill Brace Shop Inc.,). Used with permission.

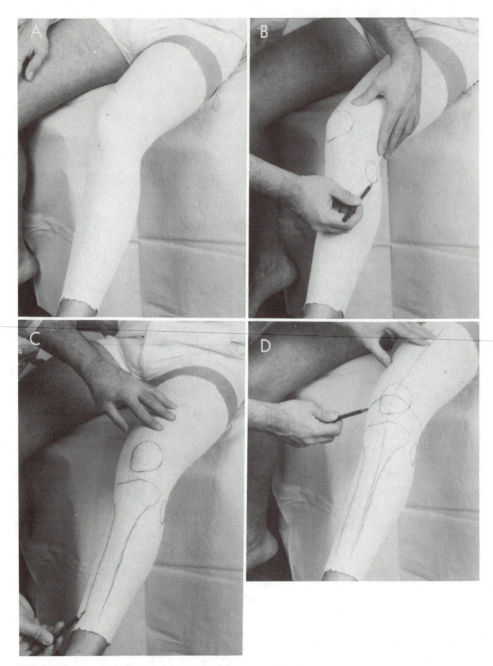

FIG 5–22.
Lenox Hill derotation brace (plaster model). **A,** apply a 4-in. stockinette to the extended leg (full extension requested but not necessary for casting). **B,** with a moistened indelible pencil, outline the patella and fibular head. **C,** outline the tibia. **D,** make vertical and transverse lines through the knee center. *(Continued.)*

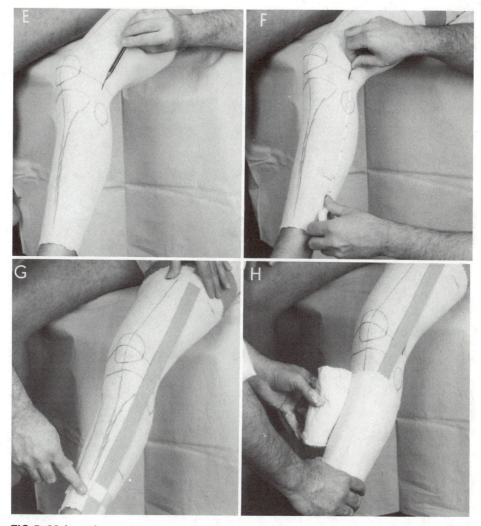

FIG 5–22 (cont.).
E, bisect the transverse line, laterally and medially. **F,** mark 8 in. above and 8 in. below the center of the knee. Cast *must* be at least this length. **G,** apply a 1-in. cutting strip lateral to the patella (with webbing, felt, or your choice of materials). **H,** wrap with *plaster* bandage (not synthetic). For the average leg, two rolls of 6 in. bandage and one roll of 4 in. bandage should suffice. *(Continued.)*

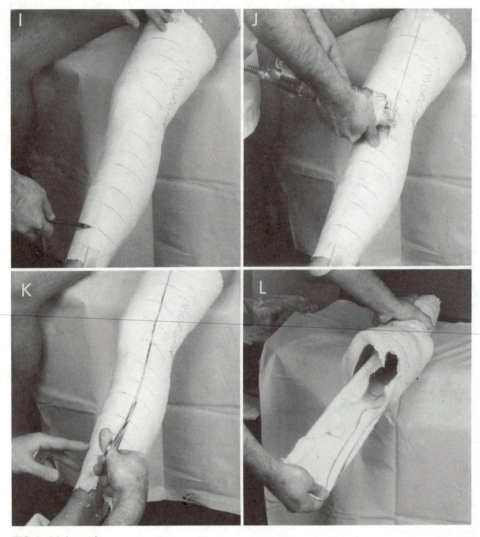

FIG 5–22 (cont.).
I, write patient's name on cast. Make a series of horizontal lines over the site of the cutting strip. **J,** univalve the cast. **K,** remove cutting strip and cut the stockinette. **L,** spring the cast off the leg; remove and discard the stockinette (if indelible pencil was *not* used, leave the stockinette in cast). *(Continued.)*

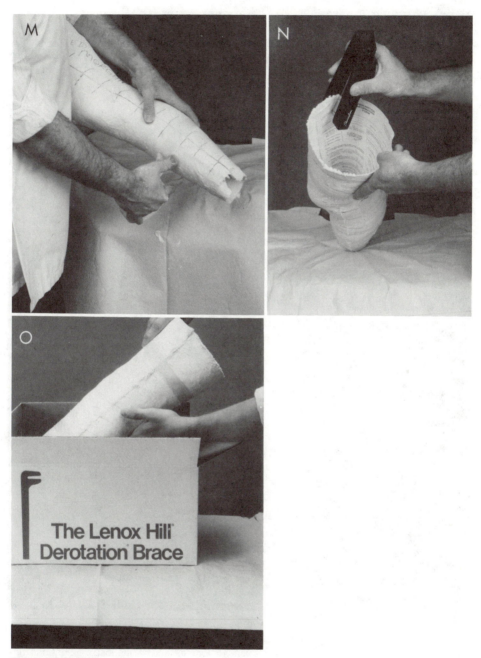

FIG 5–22 (cont.).

M, tape closed and cut the cast back to 8 in. marks (refer to **F**). **N,** complete the prescription form and staple it and other paperwork inside the cast. **O,** fill in and around the cast with packing material to protect in shipment. Place in resusable carton from the last brace delivery.

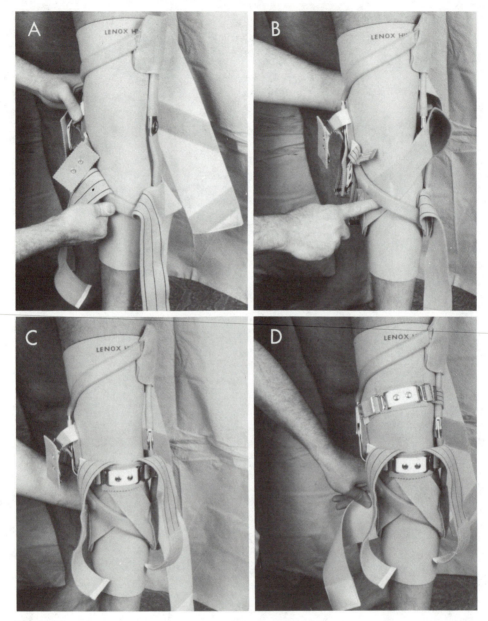

FIG 5–23.
Lenox Hill derotation brace—application instructions. **A,** align the axis of the brace with the anatomical axis. On those few braces prescribed for varus (lateral instability), the long, straight bar runs along the inside of the knee. **B,** place the medial derotation strap under the pretibial bar. Some braces may be prescribed that have only one derotation brace. **C,** cross the lateral derotation strap over the medial strap and secure with the distal patella pad. *(Continued.)*

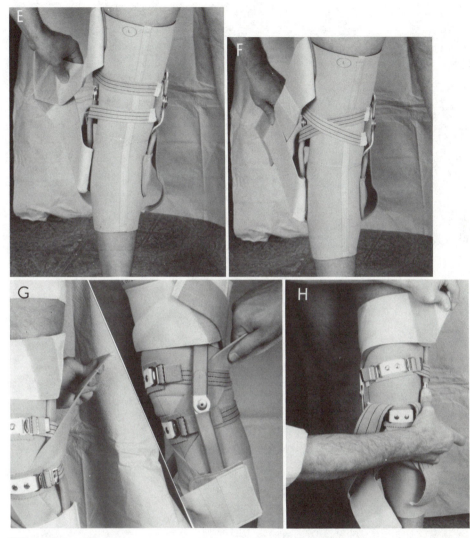

FIG 5–23 (cont.).
E, posterior view of patellar straps, shown parallel. **F,** patellar straps may also be crossed as shown.
G, patellar straps are fastened *over* the lateral upright. They can, however, be fastened under the
upright as shown at right. **H,** fasten the rubberized thigh strap while maintaining posterior pressure
on the lateral upright to prevent the brace from rotating. *(Continued.)*

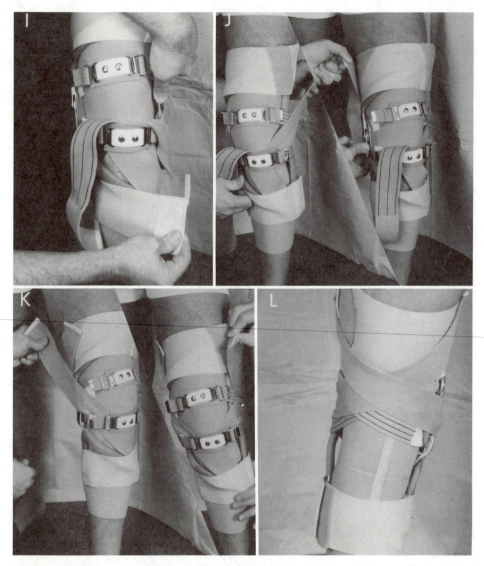

FIG 5–23 (cont.).
I, fasten the rubberized calf strap, applying pressure as described in **H. J,** spiral the medial derotation strap over the lateral upright and around to the Velcro on the medial side of the thigh strap.
K, spiral the lateral derotation strap over the medial condyle pad and around the Velcro on the lateral side of the thigh strap. **L,** the posterior view of the brace with all of the straps fastened. *(Continued.)*

6. Patella straps may also be crossed as shown (Fig 5–23,F).
7. The patella straps are fastened *over* the lateral upright. They can however be fastened under the upright as shown at right (Fig 5–23,G).
8. Fasten the rubberized thigh strap while maintaining posterior pressure on the lateral upright in order to prevent the brace from rotating (Fig 5–23,H).

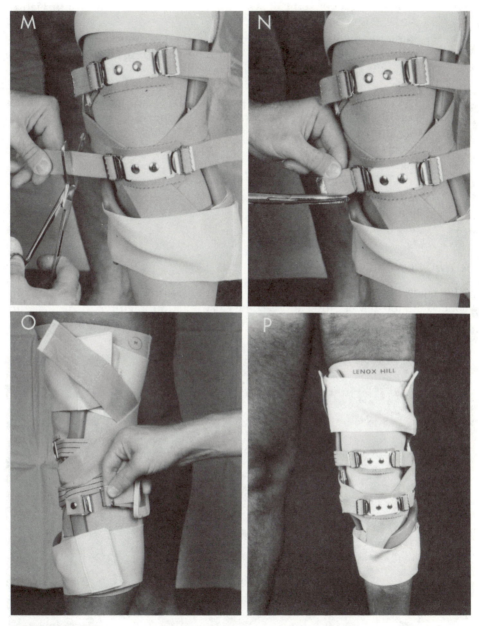

FIG 5–23 (cont.).
M, trim the patellar straps after tightening them, leaving approximately 1.5 in. **N,** clamp the metal tips (provided with instructions) onto the trimmed ends. **O,** buckle the hyperextension strap securely. This strap is only supplied with extension blocks of 10 degrees or more and with the "limited motion" attachment (or on request). **P,** the Lenox Hill derotation brace.

9. Fasten the rubberized calf strap applying pressure as shown in Figure 5–23,G (Fig 5–23,I).
10. Spiral the medial derotation strap over the lateral upright and around to the Velcro on the medial side of the thigh strap (Fig 5–23,J).
11. Spiral the lateral derotation strap over the medial condyle pad and around the Velcro on the lateral side of the thigh strap (Fig 5–23,K).
12. The posterior view of the brace with all the straps fastened (Fig 5–23,L).
13. Trim the patella after tightening them, leaving approximately 1.5 in. (Fig 5–23,M).
14. Clamp the metal tips (provided with instruction) to the trimmed ends (Fig 5–23,N).
15. Buckle the hyperextension strap securely. This strap is only supplied with extension blocks of 10 degrees or more and with the "limited motion" attachment (or upon request) (Fig 5–23,O). The Lenox Hill derotation brace (Fig 5–23,P).

DYNASPLINT

The Dynasplint brace is a recently developed spring-tension, low-load, prolonged-stretch device. Indications for its use include fractures, neurologic impairment, joint arthroplasties and arthrotomies, rheumatoid arthritis, hemo-

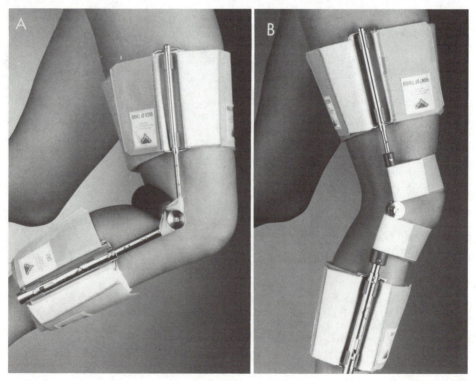

FIG 5–24.
A, Dynasplint brace for knee flexion (50 to 140 degrees of flexion). **B,** Dynasplint brace for knee extension (65 degrees of flexion to 0+ degrees extension).

philia, and tendon and ligament repairs. The concept behind the device is that prolonged stretching at moderate tension results in significant increase of motion about a contracted joint over that achieved by intense short-duration stretching.[11] For the knee there is both a flexion and an extension Dynasplint. The knee flexion splint covers from 50 degrees of flexion to 140 degrees of flexion (Fig 5–24,A). The extension splint covers from 65 degrees of flexion to 0+ degrees of extension (Fig 5–24,B).

Ordering Information

To order, contact your local authorized Dynasplint dealer, call 1-800-638-6771, or contact Dynasplint Systems Inc., 6655 Amberton Drive, Suite A, Baltimore, MD 21227.

REFERENCES

1. Bergfeld J: First, second and third degree sprains. *Am J Sports Med* 1979; 7(3):207–209.
2. Campbell DE, Glenn W: Rehabilitation of knee flexor and knee extensor muscle strength in patients with menisectomies, ligamentous repairs, and chondromalacia. *Phys Ther* 1982; 62:10–15.
3. Curl WW, Markey KL, Mitchell WA: Agility training following anterior cruciate ligament reconstruction. *Clin Orthop* 1983; 172:133–136.
4. Hastings DE: The nonoperative management of collateral ligament injuries of the knee joint. *Clin Orthop* 1980; 147:22–28.
5. Hoppenfeld S: Physical examination of the knee, in Hoppenfeld S (ed): *Physical Examination of the Spine and Extremities*. New York, Appleton-Century-Crofts, 1976, pp 171–196.
6. Indelicato PA: Nonoperative treatment of complete tears of the medial collateral ligaments of the knee. *J Bone Joint Surg Am* 1983; 65:323–329.
7. Jackson DW, Feagin JA: Quadriceps contusions in young athletes. *J Bone Joint Surg Am* 1973; 55:95–105.
8. McLeod WD, Blackburn TA: Biomechanics of knee rehabilitation with cycling. *Am J Sports Med* 1980; 8(3):175–180.
9. O'Connor GA: Collateral ligament injuries of the joint. *Am J Sports Med* 1979; 7(3):209–210.
10. O'Donaghue DM: Injuries of the knee, in O'Donaghue DH (ed): *Treatment of Injuries to Athletes*. Philadelphia, WB Saunders Co, 1984, pp 447–600.
11. Richard RL: Use of the Dynasplint to correct elbow flexion burn contracture. *J Burn Care Rehab* 1986; 7:150–152.
12. Savastano AA: Rehabilitation of the knee following surgery or injury: Restoration of function requires careful postoperative or posttraumatic management. *RI Med J* 1977; 60:569–573.
13. Steadman JR: Nonoperative measures for patellofemoral problems. *Am J Sports Med* 1979; 7(6):374–375.
14. Steadman JR: Rehabilitation of acute injuries of the anterior cruciate ligament. *Clin Orthop* 1983; 172: 129–132.
15. Steadman JR: Rehabilitation of first and second degree sprains of the medial collateral ligament. *Am J Sports Med* 1979; 7(5):300–302.
16. Yocum LA, Bachman DC, Noble HB, et al: The deranged knee: Restoration of function. A protocol for rehabilitation of the injured knee. *Am J Sports Med* 1978; 6(2):51–53.

CHAPTER 6

The Hip

INJURY: HIP POINTER
Problem: Pain

Hip pointers are contusions from direct blows to the rim of the iliac crest.[1] Symptoms include tenderness, swelling, and severe pain with a contraction or stretching of the external oblique muscle.[2]

Early treatment is important to reduce bleeding and swelling. Cold and compression should be applied. Ice packs can be used frequently. An elastic wrap may provide mild support.

INJURY: STRAIN/AVULSION OF MUSCLE

Muscle strain at the insertion into the iliac crest is characterized by pain and tenderness with contraction of the abdominal muscles. Active abduction or thigh extension will cause pain when either the gluteal or tensor fascia femoris attachments or lateral abdominal muscles are involved. Iliac crest apophysitis is also a common problem in adolescent track athletes. Stress reactions and inflammatory responses of the iliac apophysis can be caused by repetitive contractions of oblique abdominal muscles, the gluteus medius, and tensor fascia lata on the iliac apophysis.

Treatment of lesions at the iliac apophysis should include rest and the application of cold (see Chapters 1 and 12). Padding should be used for protection. Rest should continue until active motion is pain-free. Rehabilitation should be done within a pain-free range of motion. Specific exercises are described following the section on groin injuries.

INJURY: STRAINS TO THE ISCHIAL AREA

Structures in this area that are subject to strain are the origins of (1) the long head of the biceps femoris and (2) the semitendinosus on the tuberosity of the ischium. The mechanism of injury is forceful hip flexion while the knee is in extension. The muscle attachment can either be irritated or completely avulsed. Flexion of the thigh with the knee extended, active forceful contraction of the biceps muscle, and pressure over the ischial tuberosity will all cause pain.

Rest is usually sufficient[2]; however, avulsion with significant displacement may require surgical reduction of the fragment. Rehabilitation will be necessary following either surgical or nonsurgical treatment. Exercises are described following the next section on groin injuries.

INJURY: GROIN STRAINS

Groin injuries are common athletic injuries. Overuse or overexertion without sufficient warm-up can result in strains to the adductor group, iliopsoas, or rectus femoris.[2, 3] Bursitis is another problem that often affects this area.

INJURY: ADDUCTOR MUSCLE STRAINS (SARTORIUS, ADDUCTOR MAGNUS/BREVIS/LONGUS)

Violent external rotation with the thigh in abduction can result in strain to the adductor longus muscle.[2] Often adductor injuries can occur when two players kick a ball at the same time, when individuals make gliding tackles or sharp turns, or accelerates rapidly.[3]

Problem: Pain

Adductor strains are characterized by tenderness along the edge of the ramus and pain with adduction against manual resistance.[2] Pain can be felt at the muscle origin and can radiate along the medial aspect of the thigh, as well as travel toward the rectus abdominus.[3] Incomplete disruptions or second-degree strains are characterized by a stabbing pain in the groin area, hemorrhage, and local swelling a few days after injury. Complete disruptions of the muscle are characterized by an inability to contract the muscle. Renstrom and Peterson describe the "pain cycle" that develops when the individual does not abstain from activity. It occurs when activity continues despite pain, leading to further tissue damage, inflammation, and, thus, continued pain.[3]

The adductor longus can be avulsed at times, in which case symptoms will be more severe. Ruptures are often characterized by the presence of a firm mass, which is obvious when the thigh is adducted against resistance. In addition, small avulsion fractures occur at the pubic insertion of the adductors. They can cause chronic pain for weeks or months and should be suspected in groin strains that don't resolve in a few weeks.

Acute cases can be treated with ice, compression, elevation, and rest. In addition, an elastic wrap is helpful in providing support. If the injury develops into a chronic case, rest should be used until local tenderness has disappeared, and adduction against resistance is painless. Surgery may be advocated for chronic cases. Rehabilitation of the adductors is required before activity is resumed. This can consist of isometric exercises followed by dynamic training with increasing resistance, then stretching, and, finally, specialized training. Training should be tailored to the needs of the individual.[3] The groin stretching and strengthening exercises are described below.

REHABILITATION

The groin and hamstring exercises that should follow the immobilization period for the above series of injuries are as follows:

Groin Stretch

In a sitting position, with the back straight, bend the knees, place the bottom of the feet together and pull the feet toward the groin (Fig 6–1,A). Place the hands on the knees and push the knees toward the floor (Fig 6–1,B). Hold this stretch for 10 seconds. Relax, then repeat five to ten times.

Lunge Groin Stretch

Step forward with the left foot, leaving the right foot firmly planted on the ground. Bend the left knee, keep the right leg straight, and feel the stretch in the right leg (Fig 6–2,A). To increase the stretch, bend the left leg more, stepping further forward if necessary. Relax and repeat five to ten times (Fig 6–2,B). Repeat this stretch for the right leg as well.

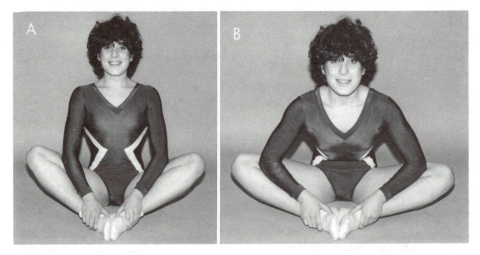

FIG 6–1.
A, the starting position for the groin stretch. Sit on the floor and place the soles of the feet together. Grasp the ankles with the hands and rest the elbows on knees. **B,** the groin stretch. Press down on the knees with the elbows until a stretch is felt in the groin. Hold this position for 10 seconds. Relax and repeat.

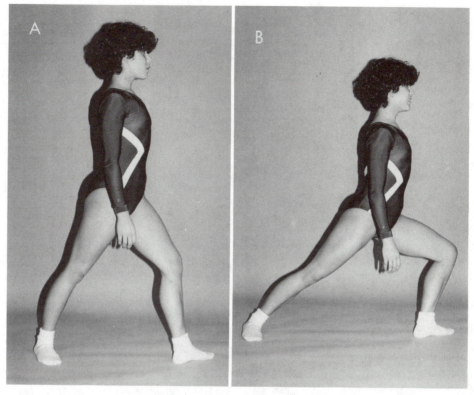

FIG 6–2.
A, the initial phase of the lunge stretch. Begin standing with both feet together, then step forward with the left leg. Bend the left leg slightly. **B,** the lunge stretch. Step farther forward with the left leg, bending it and lunging forward until there is a stretch in the groin area of the right leg. Hold the stretch for 6 to 10 seconds, relax and repeat.

Groin and Hamstring Stretch

Step to the right with the foot, about 3 to 4 ft, leaving the left foot firmly planted on the ground. The toes on the right foot should remain pointing forward. Those on the left foot will point upward during the stretching phase. Bend the right leg, keeping the left leg straight, and feel the stretch in the left leg. To increase the stretch, bend the right leg more, lowering the buttocks to the floor. Relax and repeat five to ten times. Repeat this stretch for the right leg as well.

Straddle Groin and Hamstring Stretch

Sit on the floor in a straddle position, with the legs straight and the toes toward the ceiling (Fig 6–3,A). Lean forward to the center until there is a stretch in the groin area (Fig 6–3,B). If possible, reach farther forward and try to touch the chest to the floor (Fig 6–3,C). Hold each stretch for 10 seconds. Relax. Repeat this exercise five to ten times.

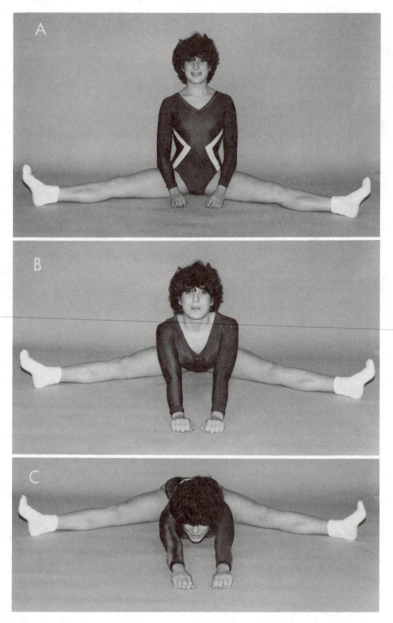

FIG 6–3.
A, the starting position for the straddle stretch. Sit on the floor with the legs straddled. Keep the back and legs straight. **B,** the straddle stretch. Lean forward to the center until a stretch is felt. Try to keep the back straight. Hold the stretch for 10 seconds. Relax. Repeat. **C,** the straddle stretch with the chest to the floor. If possible, continue leaning foward from position in **B** and try to touch the chest to the floor. *(Continued.)*

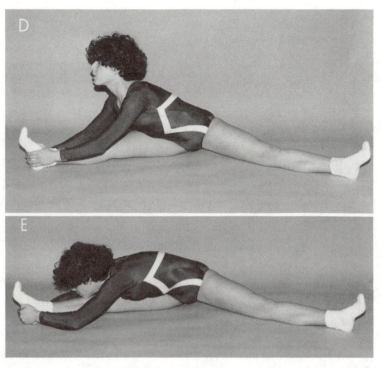

FIG 6–3 (cont.).
D, the straddle stretch to the right side. Sit on the floor and straddle the legs, as in **A.** With the toes pointing toward the ceiling and the legs straight, grasp one leg with both hands, and lean forward until a stretch is felt. Try to keep the back straight, and concentrate on trying to touch the chest to the knee. Hold this for 10 seconds, relax, repeat. Repeat this stretch leaning to the opposite side. **E,** the straddle stretch to the right with the chest to the knee.

Side Straddle Groin and Hamstring Stretch

Beginning in a straddle position as described above, lean to the right and try to grasp the right foot or midcalf (Fig 6–3,D). Try to lower the chest to the knee (Fig 6–3,E). Hold the stretch for 10 seconds. Relax and repeat five to ten times. Repeat for the left side.

Standing Straddle Groin and Hamstring Stretch

Stand in a straddle position, with the feet 1 to 2 ft apart (Fig 6–4,A). Keep the legs straight and bend forward at the waist until there is a stretch in the buttocks and back of the thighs (Fig 6–4,B). Next, bend forward farther and try to touch the palms to the floor (Fig 6–4,C). Hold each stretch for 10 seconds. Relax and repeat the exercise five to ten times.

Standing Hamstring and Calf Stretch

In a standing position keep both legs straight, feet spread slightly. Bend over at the waist and reach down to the floor until a stretch is felt behind the knees. Attempt to touch the floor or grasp the ankles. If this is not possible, grasp the

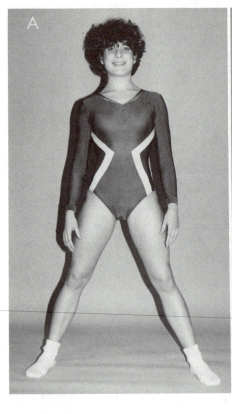

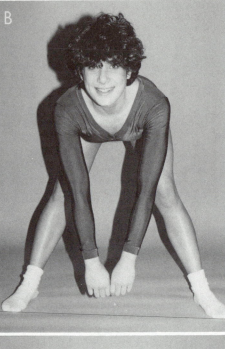

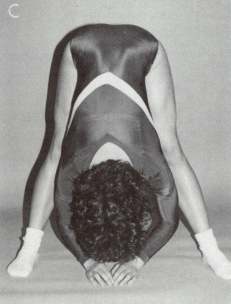

FIG 6–4.
A, the starting position for the standing straddle stretch. Stand with the feet separated, about 2 ft apart. **B,** hamstring straddle stretch. Bend forward from the hips, keeping the knees and back straight, and feel the stretch in the back of the thighs. Hold for 10 seconds. Relax and repeat. **C,** the hamstring straddle stretch with palms touching the floor. If possible, continue lowering upper body from the position shown in **B** and attempt to touch the palms to the floor. If this is not possible, attempt to grasp the ankles or the legs at midcalf.

leg at midcalf (see Figs 5–12,A and B). Hold this stretch for 10 seconds. Relax and repeat five to ten times (see also Figs 5–13,A and B for a variation of this exercise).

Hamstring Stretch

Lie supine on the floor and bend the right leg so that the sole of the shoe is on the floor. Keeping the left knee straight, raise the left leg until there is a stretch behind the knee. Hold the stretch for 10 seconds. Relax and repeat five to ten times. The hands can be used for support (Fig 6–5).

Sitting Hamstring Stretch

Sit on the floor with both legs extended straight ahead (Fig 6–6,A). Bend forward at the hips until there is a stretch behind the knees. Attempt to touch the toes, or grasp the legs at midcalf, keeping both knees straight (Fig 6–6,B). Hold the stretch position for 10 seconds. Relax and repeat five to ten times. If possible, lean forward and touch the chest to the knees (Fig 6–6,C).

Hamstring Stretch

In a standing position, place one leg on an object or surface that is higher than the waist. Keep both legs straight. Try to grasp the ankle of the elevated leg and attempt to touch the nose to the knee. Repeat for the opposite leg. Hold each stretch for 10 seconds. Repeat this exercise five to ten times.

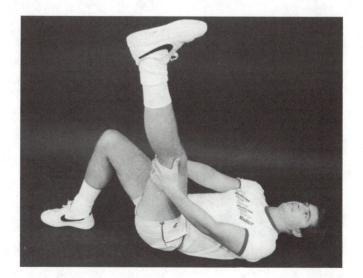

FIG 6–5.
Single hamstring stretch (supine). Lie supine on the floor. Bend the right leg so that the sole of the foot is flat on the floor. Keeping the left leg straight, flex the left hip until there is a stretch in the back of the thigh and behind the knee. Hold the stretching position for 6 to 10 seconds. Relax and repeat. The hands can be used for support and to help create a greater stretch. Repeat for the opposite leg.

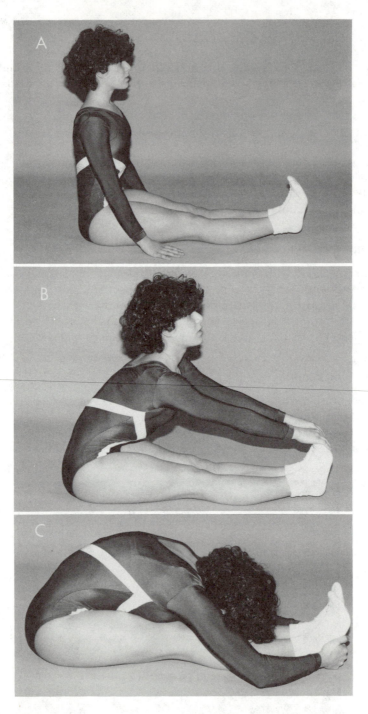

FIG 6–6.
A, the starting position for the hamstring stretch. Sit on the floor with the legs together and extended straight ahead. Sit up straight. **B,** the double hamstring stretch. Bend forward from the hips and attempt to touch the toes. Keep both legs straight. There will be a stretch in the back of the thighs and knees. If it is not possible to reach the toes, grasp the ankles or calves. Hold the stretch for 6 to 10 seconds. Relax and repeat. **C,** the double hamstring stretch with the chest to the knees. If possible, grasp the soles of the feet with both hands, and stretch forward as far as possible, so that the chest and nose touch the knees. Hold the stretch for 6 to 10 seconds. Relax and repeat.

Hamstring Hurdler's Stretch

Sit down in a hurdler's position with one leg extended forward and the other leg bent. Lean forward, attempting to grasp the ankle and touch the nose to the knee. This position stretches the hamstring muscles. Hold the stretch for 5 to 10 seconds. Relax and repeat five to ten times (see Fig 5–14,A-C).

Strengthening Exercises

Groin (Abduction).—Sitting with the legs over the edge of a table, spread the legs 12 in. apart. Attach a strap around the thighs just above the knees. Try to spread the legs apart. Apply maximum pressure for 6 seconds. Relax and repeat ten times. Do not hold your breath while doing this exercise (see Fig 5–4).

Groin (Adduction).—Sitting as in the previous exercise, place a ball between the knees. Squeeze the legs together for 6 seconds. Relax and repeat ten times. Do not hold your breath while doing this exercise (see Fig 5–5).

Knee Flexion.—Knee flexion exercises can be performed to improve hamstring strength with either free weights, Universal gym equipment, or Nautilus machines.

Nautilus Knee Flexion Machine.—Begin in the prone position. Slowly pull both heels toward the buttocks. Hold for 2 seconds. Then slowly return to the count of four to the starting position. When using a weight shoe, begin in a standing position. Lift lower leg so that the heel touches the buttocks. Hold for 2 seconds. Then slowly lower leg (see Figs 5–9,A and B). Refer to Chapter 5 for instructions on the amount of weight, number of repetitions, and frequency of lifting for this exercise.

Hip Extension.—Hip extension exercises can be performed while either standing or lying supine. Progression can be made to the Nautilus hip and back machine.

Leg Lifts (Hip Extension, Standing).—While standing, extend the right leg behind, keeping it straight. Hold this position for 10 seconds. Relax and repeat ten times (Fig 6–7,A).

Leg Lifts (Hip Extension).—Lie supine on a table or on the floor. Raise the right leg off the table, and hold for 10 seconds. Relax and repeat ten times (Fig 6–7,B).

Leg Lifts (Hip Abduction, Standing).—While standing, abduct the right leg away from the body, keeping the leg straight. Hold for 10 seconds. Relax and repeat ten times (Fig 6–7,C).

Nautilus Hip and Back Machine.—Lie supine in the machine, and place both legs over the rollers. Slide down until the hips are aligned with the cams of the machine, and grasp the handles to either side (Fig 6–8,A). Extend both

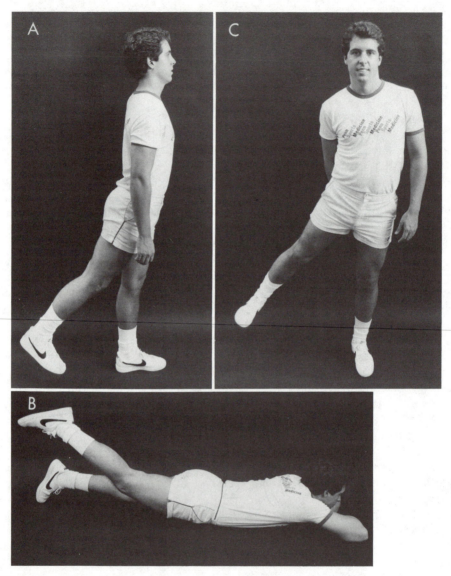

FIG 6–7.
A, the hip extension exercise. While standing, extend the injured leg behind, as shown. Keep the leg straight and do not lean forward. Hold the hip in extension for 6 seconds; lower and repeat. Repeat for the opposite leg. **B,** the hip extension exercise while prone. Lie prone on a flat surface, and raise the injured leg off the ground. Hold this position for 6 seconds. Relax and repeat. Repeat this exercise for the opposite leg. **C,** the hip abduction exercise. In the standing position, abduct the leg to the side. Keep the leg straight and do not lean sideways. Hold for 6 seconds; lower and repeat. Repeat for the opposite leg.

hips until the legs are straight. Hold this position for 2 seconds (Fig 6–8,B). Hold the left leg where it is, applying resistance against the roller, and allow the right hip and leg to flex back toward the abdomen (Fig 6–8,C). Hold this position for 2 seconds. Extend the right leg against the roller until it is parallel with the left leg (see Fig 6–8,B). Hold for 2 seconds. Hold the right leg where it is, applying

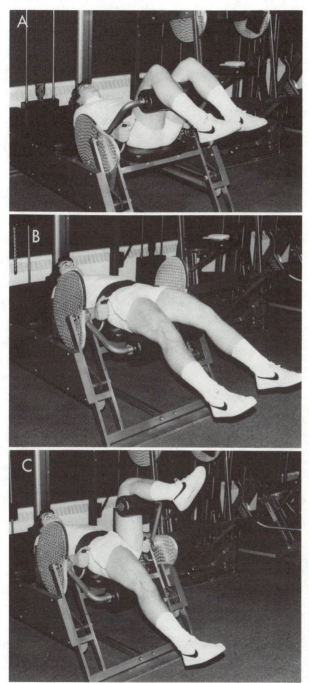

FIG 6–8.
A, the starting position for the hip and back machine. Lie supine, place the legs over the rollers as shown, and align the hips with the cams of the machine. Fasten the seat belt, and grasp the handles on either side of the hips. **B,** from position shown in **A,** extend both legs against the rollers and extend the hips as far as possible. **C,** hold the right leg in full extension and slowly flex the leg and hip. Hold for 2 seconds, then extend the leg again until it joins the right leg again. Hold both legs in extension again, then repeat for the left leg. Repeat this exercise 8 to 12 times for both legs.

resistance against the rollers, and allow the left hip and leg to flex back toward the abdomen. Hold for 2 seconds and then extend against the rollers, as done previously with the right leg, until the leg is parallel with the right. Repeat this sequence 12 times for each leg.

INJURY: HIP FLEXOR STRAINS

TENOPERIOSTITIS AND STRAIN OF THE ILIOPSOAS

The iliopsoas is a hip flexor. Repeated flexion movements, or forceful flexion of the hip against resistance, can result in strain. Weight lifting, running hills, and extensive kicking can lead to tendinitis.

Problem: Pain

The injury can be characterized by tenderness over the lesser trochanter, detectable by bimanual palpation on the medial aspect of the femur,[3] and pain with hip flexion against resistance. The "pain cycle" can develop if the rest period is not adequate.

TREATMENT

Treatment resembles that for adductor longus strains. Refer to exercise descriptions and illustrations contained in the section on strains in the ischial area.[3]

REHABILITATION

Stretching: Hip Flexion

In a standing position, flex the leg and grasp the ankle with the hand. Pull the heel as close to the buttocks as possible until a "stretch" is felt in the thigh. Hold this position for 10 seconds. Relax and repeat these exercises five to ten times (see Figs 5–15,A and B).

RECTUS FEMORIS MUSCLE AND TENDON

The rectus femoris is more susceptible to disruption than other muscles around the hip. Such injuries can occur during kicking training or repeated sprinting. Symptoms include pain above the hip joint, and pain with resisted flexion of the hip and resisted extension of the knee.

TREATMENT

Treatment resembles that for adductor longus lesions. Refer to the section on the rehabilitation of strains in the ischial area. Conservative treatment is advocated for both incomplete and complete disruptions.[3]

TENOPERIOSTITIS AND STRAIN OF THE RECTUS ABDOMINUS MUSCLE

The origins of the rectus abdominus are in close proximity with the adductor longus. Often, injury to the rectus abdominus is confused for an adductor longus injury. Injury can occur during weight lifting, goal kicking, sit-ups, pole vaulting, and tennis.

TREATMENT

Treatment resembles that for adductor longus periostitis.[3]

INJURY: BURSITIS

The hip region contains approximately 13, if not more, permanent bursae. Problems involving bursae can be either traumatic or inflammatory. Traumatic bursae contain blood caused by direct trauma.

Inflammatory bursitis can take three forms: friction, chemical, and infective. Friction bursitis develops from the tendon rubbing against the bursa. The iliopectineal bursa and trochanteric bursa are two examples of where this type of bursitis can develop.

INJURY: TROCHANTERIC BURSITIS
Problem: Inflammation and Pain

The bursa that overlies the greater trochanter can become irritated and inflamed.[1] Trochanteric bursitis is characterized by tenderness, pain, and crepitation with movement of the thigh. Hip flexion and extension, or rotation with extension, can involve sliding of the tensor fascia latae over the trochanter, which will be painful when there is inflammation. A direct blow, infection, or friction between adjacent bursal walls, are among possible contributing factors. Anatomical conditions in runners such as a broad pelvis, or leg-length discrepancy can contribute to its irritation. Rest, ice, and, occasionally, the use of steroids are recommended for treatment.

PREVENTION

Conditioning the pelvis and the lower extemities can help prevent groin injuries. Range of motion exercises against resistance and special stretching exercises should be performed. Among the muscles to target for strengthening are adductors, lower back, and abdominal muscles.

INJURY: HIP ABDUCTOR STRAINS—GLUTEUS MEDIUS STRAIN

Overuse can result in strains of the gluteus medius, and the development of chronic cases is common. Active contraction of the muscle against resistance will cause pain if the external rotators have been strained. Flexion against resistance, especially with external rotation, will be painful when the psoas muscle is injured. In addition, if a muscle has been injured, forced passive motion of its opposer will elicit pain.[2]

TREATMENT

Strains should be treated initially with ice, and then rehabilitation, including stretching exercises.

REHABILITATION

Gluteus Medius Stretch

Sit on the floor with the left leg extended straight ahead. Cross the right leg over, placing the sole of the foot flat on the floor, leaving the knee flexed and directly in front of the body (Fig 6–9). With the hip facing forward, rotate the upper body to the left. Support the weight on the right hand, and place the elbow of the left arm against the right leg, applying pressure for 10 seconds. Relax and repeat ten times. Repeat in the opposite direction.

Straight Leg Raises
Isometric Straight Leg Lifts.—Follow the steps given below.

1. Begin in a supine position, with the legs fully extended (see Fig 5–1,A).
2. With the leg straight, lift the leg so that the heel is 12 in. off the floor. The toe of the foot should be pulled toward the knee so that they are pointed toward the ceiling.
3. Hold the leg in this position for a full 10 seconds (see Fig 5–1,B).
4. After 10 seconds, lower the leg and repeat the exercise with the opposite leg.
5. Continue to alternate legs until you have done 30 lifts on each leg. This program should be done *two* times a day.

Don't expect results in two or three days. It usually takes three to four weeks before there is any noticeable improvement. Be patient and do the exercises faithfully.

Isometric Straight Leg Raises With Weights.—Repeat the above leg lifts, holding each raise for 2 to 3 seconds. Complete three sets of ten leg raises with

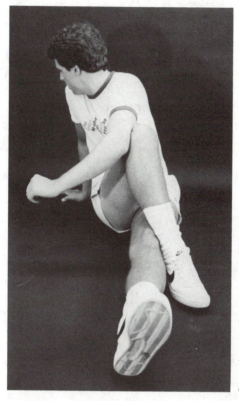

FIG 6–9.
The gluteus medius stretch. Sit on the floor. Flex the right leg and cross it over the left leg, placing the sole of the foot on the floor as shown. Rotate the upper body to the right, keeping the hips square and the buttocks on the floor. Place the left elbow on the side of the knee as shown. Apply gentle pressure to the leg with the elbow. There should be a stretch in the right buttock and hip. Hold the stretch for 10 seconds. Relax and repeat. Repeat on the opposite side.

a 30-second rest between each set. When the 30 leg lifts become easy to do add 2.5 lb to the ankle and exercise with that weight until it becomes easy. Progress with weights (2.5-lb increments) until you can master one-tenth of your total body weight. These exercises should be done at least once a day or, preferably, twice a day (every day). If soreness or irritation develops due to the exercise program, use ice for 30 minutes following each exercise session.

Quadriceps Extension Exercises

Isotonic Knee Program.—These exercises may be done on a Universal Gym Machine, a Nautilus knee extension machine, other knee extension benches, or with a York iron health shoe.

Knee extension.—Begin in a sitting position. Slowly extend the leg until it is fully extended. Hold the leg in the fully extended position for 2 seconds, then slowly lower it to the starting position (see Figs 5–6,A and B). Refer to Chapter 5 for instructions on the amount of weight to be used, frequency for the exercise, and other important information.

Hip abduction and adduction.—The exercises for hip abduction and adduction are described in the rehabilitation section following the discussion of groin strains (see Figs 5–4 and 5–5).

Hip flexion exercises.—In a standing position, lift the leg up and bend the knee, as if stepping up on a stool. Hold this position for 6 seconds. Relax and repeat ten times (see Fig 5–8).

REFERENCES

1. Kulund DN: The torso, hip and thigh, in Kulund DN (ed): *The Injured Athlete.* Philadelphia, JB Lippincott Co, 1982, pp 331–360.
2. O'Donaghue DH: Injuries of the pelvis and hip, in O'Donaghue DH (ed): *Treatment of Injuries to Athletes.* Philadelphia, WB Saunders Co, 1984, pp 407–432.
3. Renstrom PA, Peterson L: Groin injuries in athletes. *Br J Sports Med* 1980; 14:30–36.

CHAPTER 7

The Low Back

INJURIES: SPRAINS, STRAINS, AND STABLE FRACTURES

Ligamentous sprains and muscular strains are, in fact, infrequent causes of low back pain in the athlete. The same can be said for nondisplaced, stable fractures of the vertebral body, transverse processes, spinous processes, and neural arches. With regard to these injuries, treatment basically consists of rest, support, and application of ice in acute phase, followed by moist heat in the subcutaneous phase. With conservative management these injuries heal without residual disability. However, appropriate rehabilitative exercises are indicated to effect maximum recovery.

INJURY: SPONDYLOLYSIS

Spondylolysis, a stress reaction/fracture involving the pars interarticularis, is the major cause of lower back pain among young athletes. The problem is most frequently seen in pole vaulters, gymnasts, interior linemen, swimmers, and divers. In a study performed by Jackson,[9] 11 of 100 female gymnasts had bilateral L-5 pars interarticularis defects, a frequency much higher than that reported for female nonathletic counterparts.[9, 11]

Spondylolysis may be asymptomatic or symptomatic.[5] Clinical diagnosis is strongly suggested when the following can be identified: (1) pain localized to the area of the posterior superior iliac spine; (2) hamstring spasm; (3) loss of normal lumbar lordosis; and (4) limitation of extension of the lumbar spine.

Hyperextension is thought to be a predominant mechanism contributing to the development of this injury. Jackson et al.[9] reported that their experience indicates that football, karate, gymnastics, hurdling, pole-vaulting, high jump, and other "jarring sports"[9, 11] result in a higher incidence of pars defects. Spondylolysis is not limited to these activities, and can develop in those participating in less vigorous sports, as well as in nonathletes.[9]

Spondylolysis patients can also be divided into two groups: (1) preroentgenographic, those with normal roentgenograms and abnormal bone scans and (2) roentgenographic, those with x-ray evidence of a stress fracture involving the pars. Treatment of both includes limitation of activities, the use of a Boston brace, the use of a bedboard, Williams flexion exercises, hamstring stretching, and the avoidance of hyperextension activities. Treatment, as outlined, can arrest the preroentgenographic process. Once there is radiographic evidence of stress fracture involving the pars, healing per se does not occur. Treatment will result in the relief of symptoms; however, it will not reverse established roentgenographic findings. Extension of the lumbar spine must be avoided.

Given the likelihood of spondylolysis developing in gymnasts, preventive measures are important. Goldberg[5] recommends a conditioning program that includes strengthening of the abdominal muscles, antilordotic exercises, stretching of the tight lumbosacral fascia, and stretching of the hamstring muscles. The exercises include pelvic tilts, both recumbent and upright, and sit-ups, both partial sit-ups with the hips and knees flexed, and side-lying sit-ups for the lateral abdominal muscles.[5]

INJURY: JUVENILE DISK/HERNIATED NUCLEUS PALPOSUS

Juvenile disk, or herniated nucleus palposus, in children and adolescents is a rare phenomenon[3, 4, 12, 19] and follows a different clinical course than that occurring in adults. Bradford and Garcia[3] report that the incidence of surgery is low. Accurate diagnoses may not be made or may be delayed because individuals may have pain only in the leg and not in the back.[2-4, 12, 19]

The level of the lesion in children is usually at L-5/S-1 or L-4/L-5.[3, 8, 12]

The signs and symptoms that characterize herniated disks in children and adolescents have been purported to be different from those experienced by adults.[2] Bradford and Garcia[3] reviewed the opinions of several authors on this matter. While some authors identify pain as the predominant symptom for young individuals, others report physical signs and objective findings.[3] Borgesen and Vang[2] cite Sprangfort on the relation between the Lasègue's sign and age; the sign tends to be higher in the younger populations. The reflex changes, and the sensory and motor defects that occur in the adult population are noted to be less frequent in individuals under 20 years of age.[2, 19] Winter[19] attributes this to greater resiliency in the nerve roots of children, and Bradford and Garcia[3] and Borgesen and Vang[2] refer to a greater amount of mobility in the young. The issue of the difference of the nature of this injury in adults and children is not indisputable. Several other authors do not believe that there is a significant difference between the two age groups.[3, 4]

Signs and symptoms characterizing the problem in this age group include low back pain with radiation into a lower extremity,[3, 4, 12, 19] restriction of lumbar motion,[4] lumbar fixation,[3] positive Lasègue's test,[3] sciatic scoliosis, positive straight leg raising,[3, 4, 19] sensory changes involving the L-5 and S-1 dermatome,[3, 12, 19] gait abnormalities,[3, 4] decreases in ankle jerk,[3, 4, 12] changes in the lordotic lumbar angle,[3, 4] sciatica,[3, 4] and paresthesia.[4] Lorenz and McCulloch[12] reported a 50% or more reduction in straight leg raising, and pain in the lower limb as a predominant symptom.

Antecedent trauma has been reported to be a significant etiological factor, with incidence reported to be 30% to 60% of cases,[3] which is comparable to that reported for adult cases.[3] Degeneration is a second possible etiological factor and Borgesen and Vang[2] propose that it is the primary cause, and view trauma as a precipitating factor.

With regards to conservative treatment, most authors recommend bed rest[3, 4, 19] the use of a bedboard, traction,[3, 4] heat,[19] analgesics,[3, 4, 19] and medication in the acute phase, and exercises[3, 4] and the use of a lumbosacral corset in the subacute phase. Our experience has been that an acute herniated nucleous palposus in adolescents requires surgery, the problem not being amenable to conservative means. Thus, when conservative treatment proves to be ineffective, surgical means are required. Among methods reported in the literature are (1) chemonucleolysis, (2) laminectomy,[4, 12] (3) laminectomy with fusion,[3] and (4) hemilaminectomy without spinal fusion.[3, 4, 19] Seventy-three percent to 98% of those children who undergo diskectomy after conservative treatment had failed are reported to have successful results.[12]

INJURY: IDIOPATHIC LOW BACK PAIN

In addition to spondylolysis and disk disease, some individuals suffer from what may be described as, for lack of a better name, idiopathic low back pain.

In Howell's study[6] of 17 light-weight women rowers, 82% of the population reported having occasional or chronic low backache or discomfort. Ninety-four percent of the rowers were classified as hyperflexible in a test of upper and lower back motion and hamstring length. Hyperflexion motion of the lumbar spine was observed in 76%.

The correlation between the incidence of low back pain, and both hyperflexion motion and adherence to a regular stretching program, was high.[6] The authors recommend that each rower be tested to identify loose or tight muscles and motions, and instructed to avoid stretching these muscles.[6]

The longer chronic pain goes untreated, the less successful rehabilitative measures have been. Of patients who went untreated for six months, 30% returned to function, compared to only 10% of those who went untreated for a year.[15]

TREATMENT

Exercises have been recommended for the treatment of idiopathic low back pain by a series of authors. Kendall and Jenkins[10] compared the effects of (1) mobility and exercise; (2) lumbar isometric flexion exercises; and (3) hyperextension exercises on idiopathic low back pain. Those who performed isometric flexion exercises experienced remission at a statistically significant rate compared to other groups. They conclude that isometric flexion exercises are a safe and effective approach to the treatment of low back pain.

Claudia Jackson and Mark Brown and others[7, 8] stress the role of exercise

(1) in decreasing pain; (2) in strengthening muscles; (3) in decreasing mechanical stress; (4) in improving fitness level; (5) in stabilizing the hypermobile segments; (6) in improving posture; and (7) in improving mobility.

Exercise to Decrease Pain.—Exercise is designated by Claudia Jackson as one way to decrease pain by opening the intervertebral foramen and relieving the pressure on the nerve. While it can provide temporary relief, it will not be sufficient to effect healing and symptom reversal. Exercise is also said to decrease pain by increasing endorphin levels.[8]

Exercise to Strengthen Weak Muscles.—Patients with low back pain often demonstrate reduced trunk extensor strength, and such muscular insufficiency can contribute to idiopathic low back pain.[9] Low back exercises can be performed to strengthen the muscles in the low back region. There are several different theories as to what kind of exercise is most beneficial. The relationship between exercise and back pain is addressed in a series of articles reviewed by Jackson[7]: Pederson et al.,[18] Nachemson,[15] Berkson,[1] and others.[7]

Decrease Mechanical Stress.—Mechanical stress has been found to be related to low back pain. Proper exercise selection therefore is necessary because of the loads that certain exercises produce in the lumbar spine.[8]

Improve Fitness Level.—Increased fitness levels have been associated with lower incidence of back pain. Exercise therefore can help prevent injuries as well as lower the rate of recurrence.

Stabilize Hypermobile Segments.—Stabilization of the hypermobile segment through exercise has been hypothesized but not proved.

Improve Posture.—While many authors suggest using exercise along with postural training as a means to improve posture, there is no evidence to support this claim.[8] The studies of Danes, Fox, and Flint, cited by Jackson,[8] all failed to show an improvement in posture in individuals on either isometric flexion exercises, or isotonic abdominal strengthening exercises.

Three particular forms of exercise are normally associated with the management of low back pain: (1) flexion; (2) extension; and (3) aerobics. There is a specific function of each that helps in aiding pain.

REHABILITATION

Low Back Exercises

The following exercises, used at the University of Pennsylvania Sports Medicine Center, are designed to increase the flexibility of the low back. They must be done regularly, three to four times a day, preferably in the morning, midday, afternoon, and before bed. They should not be done forcefully; the stretch should be comfortable. Moist heat, in the form of a shower or hydrocollator packs, may be used before exercising; however, it is not essential. Each exercise should be repeated five times.

Flexion Exercises

Flexion exercises can be used to treat low back pain. They achieve four objectives:

1. Stretch the back extensors that have overdeveloped due to assumption of the upright posture.
2. Strengthen abdominal muscles and glutei.
3. Open the intervertebral foramen and facet joints to reduce compression on the nerve.
4. Free the posterior fixation of the lumbosacral articulation.

Knee Raises

Raise the knee to the chest. Hold for 5 to 10 seconds. Repeat with the opposite leg. Repeat with both legs (Figs 7–1,A through 7–1,F). This exercise strengthens the spinal extensors.[7]

Abdominal Exercises

Tighten the abdominal muscles. Try to flatten the low back against the floor; hold for 10 seconds (Fig 7–2).

Leg Raises

Raise leg, keeping knee straight. Provide assistance if necessary by grasping the ankle. Hold the stretch for 10 seconds. Repeat with the opposite leg (see Fig 6–5). In bilateral straight leg raises, abdominal activity is minimal, and there is no strengthening benefit.[9, 10]

Sit-ups (Partial/Full)

Raise the head to the chest while attempting to lift the shoulders off the floor. Hold for 4 to 6 seconds. When there has been some improvement, try to raise the upper body further from the floor (Fig 7–3).

Flexion Chair Exercises

Sit in a hard chair with feet on the floor and legs apart (Fig 7–4,A). Slowly lower the upper body between the legs until a stretch is felt in the lower back. Relax and hold the stretch (Fig 7–4,B).

Extension Exercises

Extension exercises can be performed in either the flexed or neutral position, or in a hyperextension position. The former will benefit motor recruitment, endurance, and strength, while the latter can improve spinal mobility and strengthen the extensors.[7]

Extension exercises are recommended because a significant loss of back extensor strength characterizes chronic back problems, as well as low extensor endurance.[7] Extensor strength tends to be lesser than flexor strength in a normal population.

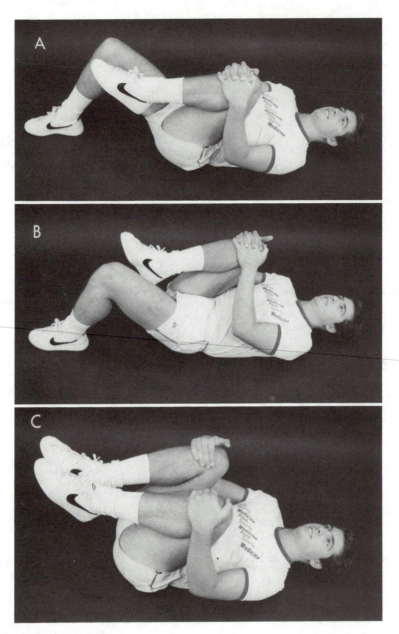

FIG 7–1.
A, the knee raise stretch with the left leg. Lie on the floor or on a table and bend both knees to 90 degrees, keeping the soles of the feet on the floor. Raise one knee to the chest, and pull it in with the hands, as shown. There should be a stretch in the lower back. Hold this position for 10 seconds. Relax and repeat. **B,** the knee raise stretch with the right leg. Repeat the exercise described in **A** with the opposite leg. **C,** the knee raise stretch using both legs. Pull both knees toward the chest, pulling gently with the hands, as shown. Keep the hips on the floor. Hold the stretching position for 10 seconds. Relax and repeat *(Continued.)*

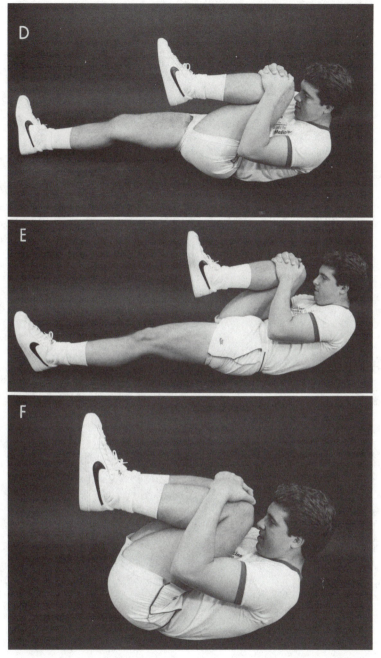

FIG 7–1 (cont.).

D, the knee raise exercise with the left leg and the head raise. Repeat the exercise as described for **A,** and in addition, raise the head off the ground and try to touch it to the knee. Begin the head raise by touching the chin to the chest first. Hold for 10 seconds. Relax and repeat. **E,** the knee raise exercise with the right leg and the head raise. Repeat the exercise as described in **B,** and, in addition, raise the head off the ground and try to touch it to the knee. Begin the head raise by touching the chin to the chest first. Hold the stretch for 10 seconds. Relax and repeat. **F,** the double knee raise with head raise. Repeat the exercise as described in **C,** and, in addition, raise the head off the ground and try to touch it to the knee. Begin the head raise by touching the chin to the chest first. Hold the stretch for 10 seconds. Relax and repeat.

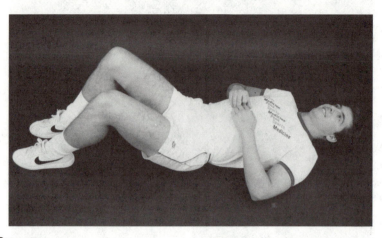

FIG 7–2.
The abdominal tightening exercise. Lie on the floor or on a table. Bend the knees to 90 degrees, keeping the soles of the feet on the floor. Tighten the abdominal muscles and attempt to flatten the lower portion of the back to the floor. Hold this position for 10 seconds. Relax and repeat.

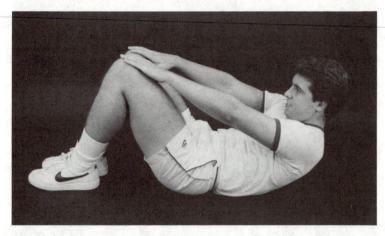

FIG 7–3.
The abdominal curl. Lie supine on a table, or on the floor. Raise the chin to the chest and lift the shoulders off the floor, reaching toward the knees with the hands. Hold the curl-up for 4 to 6 seconds. Relax and repeat.

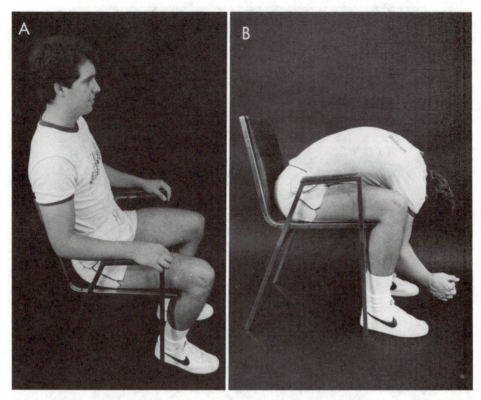

FIG 7–4.
Williams flexion chair exercises. **A,** the starting position for the flexion chair stretching exercise. Sit up straight in a chair with the feet on the floor about 12 in. apart. **B,** bend over at the waist slowly until the upper body touches, or passes between, the legs. There should be a stretch in the lower back. Hold the position for 10 seconds. Relax and repeat.

Hyperextension.—Hyperextension exercises accomplish several purposes. Among these are (1) restoration of normal lordosis through increased mobility; (2) help in reduction of nuclear pressure on the annulus; and (3) increase in strength of spinal muscles.[7] These exercises should not be prescribed for spondylolysis.

Extension to Neutral.—Patients with postural low back pain that is aggravated by prolonged sitting and flexion, patients whose work involves lifting moderate to heavy loads, and patients with possible posterior or posterolateral disk protrusion are those likely to benefit from extension exercises.[7]

The authors recomend an aerobic conditioning program as well as walking, jogging, swimming, or bicycling. Jumping rope is not recommended.[7]

Partial Arch-up.—Lie on the floor, prone, with legs straight and together, chin on the floor, and arms to sides with palms on the floor (Fig 7–5,A). Keeping the legs and hips on the floor, do a push-up–like action, lifting the head, neck, and chest off the floor. Hold for 6 seconds; lower and repeat (Fig 7–5,B).

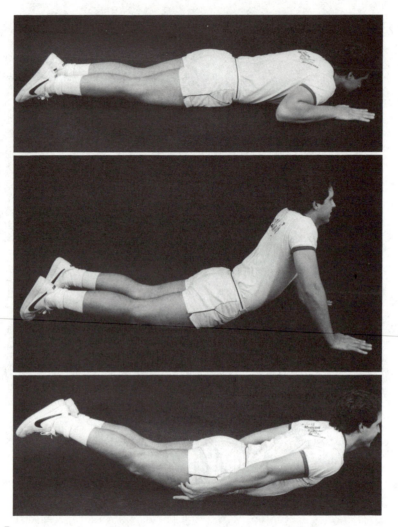

FIG 7–5.
A, the starting position for extension exercises. Lie prone with legs straight and together, chin on the floor, and arms at sides, with palms resting flat against floor. **B,** partial arch-up. Keep legs together and hips on floor, and perform half push-up, lifting head, neck, and chest off of floor. Hold for 6 seconds; lower and repeat. **C,** full arch-up. Lie prone, with legs straight and together, arms at sides, resting on floor. Arch up, lifting the head, neck, chest, and legs off floor. Hold for 6 seconds. Relax and repeat.

Full Arch-up.—Begin prone with arms resting on the floor at sides. Arch up, lifting head, neck, chest, and legs off the floor (Fig 7–5,C). Hold for 6 seconds; lower and repeat.

Nautilus Hip and Back Machine.—Lie supine in the machine and place both legs over the rollers. Slide down until the hips are aligned with the cams of the machine and grasp the handles to either side (see Fig 6–8,A). Extend both hips until the legs are straight. Hold this position for 2 seconds (see Fig 6–8,B).

Hold the left leg where it is, applying resistance against the roller, and allow the right hip and leg to flex backward toward the abdomen (see Fig 6–8,C). Hold this position for 2 seconds. Extend the right leg against the roller until it is parallel with the left leg (see Fig 6–8,B). Hold for 2 seconds. Hold the right leg where it is, applying resistance against the rollers, and allow the left hip and leg to flex back toward the abdomen. Hold for 2 seconds and then extend against the rollers, as for the right leg, until the leg is parallel with the right. Repeat this sequence 8 to 12 times for each leg. (Refer to Chapter 5 for instructions on how to use the Nautilus.)

In addition to the exercise program, the patient should obtain a bedboard made from ¾-in. plywood cut to the size of the mattress. The board should be placed between the mattress and box spring. If a bedboard is not available, the mattress should be placed on the floor.

THE MODIFIED BOSTON BRACE SYSTEM*

The development of prefabricated thermoplastic braces to aid in the treatment of spinal deformities, such as scoliosis, is recent. The first such system, the Boston brace, was introduced 10 years ago. The efficacy and high patient acceptance of these semirigid, closely fitting orthoses resulted in a reassessment of the use of back braces for spinal disorders in general.[14]

A number of back braces used in the past for a variety of back disorders have fallen into disrepute. There appears to be a number of quite different factors responsible for this, ranging from theoretical concerns about their effect on the long-term function to poor patient acceptance and compliance. These braces, which include the Norton Brown, Jewett hyperextension, and chairback braces, were commonly prescribed for back pain due to a number of different etiologies.[14]

In addition, these braces were often prescribed without concurrent exercise programs, with resultant loss of spinal motion and strength, which sometimes further exacerbated the back pain when the brace was removed. Finally, the older braces were often bulky, and had leather and metal parts with a limited number of contact sites on the torso and pelvis. Patients complained of the braces being uncomfortable; they frequently were not accepted or worn.[14]

Most of the thermoplastic orthoses developed to treat spinal deformities in children or adolescents incorporated as a design feature a forward flexion of the orthosis, designed to reduce lumbar lordosis, flatten the back, and increase the torso contact.[14]

The clinical application of this antilordotic feature of the Boston brace system soon became evident. Back pain in athletically active youngsters, although due to a variety of etiologies, including spondylolysis, apophyseal fracture, disk disease, or back strain, appeared to have as a common etiological feature hyperlordosis of the lumbar spine, either in the occurrence of injury or in its persistence.[14]

*Adapted from Micheli LJ: *B.O.B.: The Boston Overlap Brace Manual.* Avon, Mass, O&P Systems Inc., 1985.

The potential for effective treatment of back pain in athletically active children and adolescents with thermoplastic orthoses was confirmed, according to Micheli,[13] by clinical trials.[13, 14]

The original braces had posterior openings and were constructed of polypropylene with semirigid ¼-in. polyethylene liners. A number of different designs of the back brace were subsequently tried. The present unlined, anterior-opening polyethylene with reinforced spring steel—the Boston overlap brace (BOB)—is the culmination of these clinical investigations. At present, this brace is available in either polyethylene in ⅟₁₆-in., ⅛-in., or ³⁄₁₆-in. thickness, or polypropylene in ⅛-in. thickness. This brace is usually prescribed unlined. The brace is available in contours of 0, 15, or 30 degrees of lumbar lordosis.

The efficacy and high rate of acceptance of these thermoplastic braces for back pain in young athletes—particularly in spondylolysis—served as an incentive for thermoplastic bracing in a variety of other back disorders including low back pain and upper back pain in adults.

Experience with this application of thermoplastic total contact has proved promising. While this experience is more recent, and study is needed to determine the long-term efficacy and effect on the natural history of back pain in adults, the short-term observations, in and of themselves, provide an adequate basis for the continued use of this technique.[14]

For illustrations of the brace, and fitting procedures, see Figures 7–6 through 7–14 (The Boston Brace can be ordered from O&P Systems, Inc., 20 Ledin Dr., Avon, MA 02322, or by calling 1-800-262-2235.)

FIG 7–6.
The Boston Overlap Brace (BOB) is an anterior-opening, antilordotic, semilordotic, or lordotic brace constructed of an adjustable external shell, made of preformed variable-thickness special-formula thermoformed material, to which may be added an additional liner of polyethylene foam. The anterior closures are of spring steel (in 1-in. increments) from 6 to 12 in. long, shaped for the appropriate degree of concavity, and are covered by Dacron. The fasteners are of Dacron-covered Velcro, or optional cotton strapping with buckles.

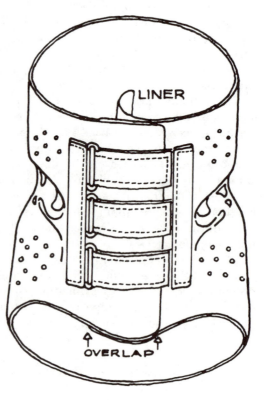

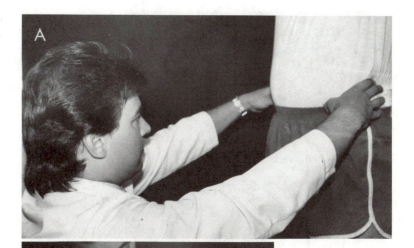

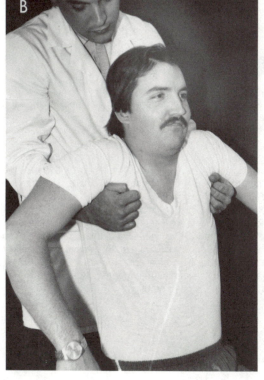

FIG 7–7.
Patient evaluation by the orthotist. **A,**
review the patient clinically. Note the
suppleness of the spine. Are the shoulders
and iliac crests level? If not, measure the
leg length for discrepancies. Are there any
prominent bony areas that must be
relieved of excessive pressure? Check the
patient's tissue tone and postural habits.
Evaluate the patient's attitude toward
bracing. Check that the iliac crests are
level; if not, equalize the leg lengths by a
shoe lift or wedge. **B,** with the patient
sitting on a stool, distract the spine by
elevating the axillae with your forearms, or
let the patient elevate himself. At the same
time, ask the patient to increase or
decrease lordosis for the most comfortable
position without pain. This is the position in
which you should fabricate your initial
brace. Any hip contractures about the
pelvis must be considered—sitting vs
standing. The iliac depression in
conjunction with total contact abdominal
compression will distract the lumbar spine.

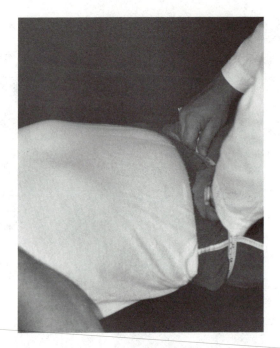

FIG 7–8.
Patient measurement and selection of an appropriate overlap brace: (1) Fashion stockinette to the appropriate width and length to cover the patient, or use a cast shirt. The stockinette over the underwear preserves the patient's modesty and provides a sense of security. (2) Eliminate wrinkles in the stockinette or cast shirt after it is applied to the patient. (3) Ask the patient to lie down on a firm table, if possible, while measurements are being taken. *Snug* circumferential measurements are taken of the hips above the pubis, the waist, and the chest below the nipple line. (4) Select the module size from the *size chart* with reference to the patient's data sheet. A smaller size may be used on an obese patient to allow for displacement of tissue and a larger size on a patient with good muscle tone, since minimal tissue displacement within a month can be expected. (5) The waist measurement is most important and should be used *first* to determine the proper module size. Because of the flexibility from which the modules are fabricated, the hip and chest circumferences can be 2 to 5 cm larger or smaller at the inferior and superior borders, i.e., the hips may be smaller while the chest is larger, or vice versa. (6) To eliminate the patient's back pain, the proper sized module should have no void areas about the waist. (7) Determine that the module selected is long enough, i.e., determine whether an "untrimmed" module should be used.

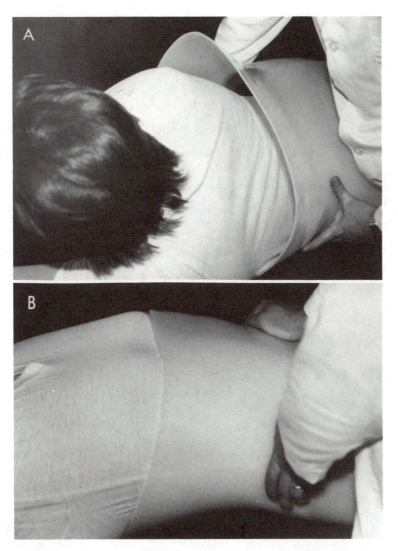

FIG 7–9.
Initial fitting. **A,** with the patient lying on one side with knees flexed slightly, slip the module around the body and position properly. The patient can now roll onto the back. **B,** exert medial force on the module with your hands and force down on the iliac crests. The anterior opening should be over-lapped not less than 2 nor more than 5 in. at top or bottom, but not both.

FIG 7–10.

Anterior inferior trim line. The anterior inferior trim line is kept as distal as the patient can tolerate. For adolescents, the added length below allows for more growth without replacing the module and prevents the soft tissues from being pinched between the symphysis pubis and the brace. The midpoint should extend over the pubis when the patient is standing. The trim lines for the thigh allow just 90 degrees of flexion for sitting on a firm chair. Depress the patient's thigh by inserting one finger between the brace and thigh when the patient is sitting in this 90 degree position to determine whether the brace fits properly.

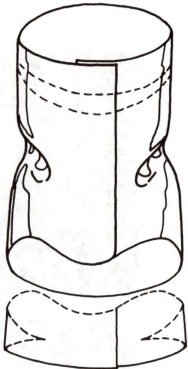

FIG 7–11.

Lateral inferior trim line. The standard lateral trim line flows from the anterior inferior line passing approximately 2 cm above the top of the greater trochanters flowing down the posterior inferior line.

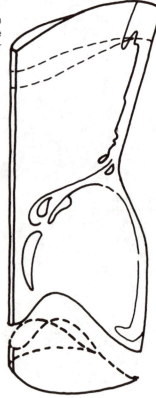

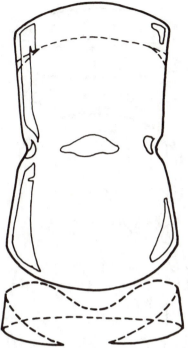

FIG 7–12.
Posterior inferior trim line. The standard posterior inferior trim line extends as low as possible, but no more than one finger from the seat of a hard chair when the patient is sitting with hips flexed at 90 degrees. Establishing this line too high will result in increased lumbar lordosis and, often, unsightly bulges of soft tissue.

FIG 7–13.
The standard anterior superior trim line is located at the base of the sternum to prevent impingement on the xiphoid process. The anterior overlap should not be less than 1½ in. nor more than 3 in. when the brace is completed; i.e., the vertical closure should be less than ¾ to ¹⁄₁₂ in. on either side of the midline when secured snugly on the patient. With the brace manually secured snugly on the patient, mark the position of the overlap by drawing a vertical line along the anterior edge of the plastic. The goal here is to achieve a final overlap that is vertical when the brace is in place on the patient.

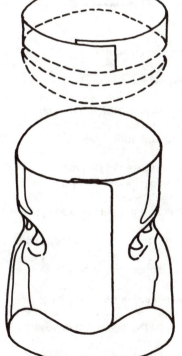

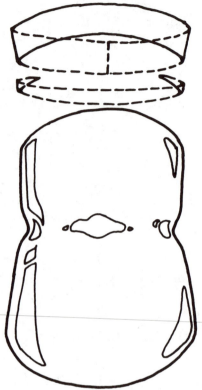

FIG 7–14.
Posterior superior. The standard posterior superior trim line originates at the level of the eighth thoracic vertebra just inferior to the scapula. This height allows for a lever arm in the reduction of excessive lumbar lordosis. The trim line flows posterolaterally to the xiphoid process anteriorly.

REFERENCES

1. Berkson M, Schultz A, Nachemson AL, et al: Voluntary strengths of male adults with acute low back syndrome. *Clin Orthop* 1977; 129:84.
2. Borgesen SE, Vang PS: Herniation of the lumbar intervertebral disc in children and adolescents. *Acta Orthop Scand* 1974; 45:540–549.
3. Bradford DS, Garcia A: Herniations of the lumbar intervertebral disk in children and adolescents: A review of 30 surgically treated cases. *JAMA* 1969; 210:2045–2051.
4. DeOrio JK, Bianco AJ: Lumbar disc excision in children and adolescents. *J Bone Joint Surg Am* 1982; 64:991–995.
5. Goldberg MJ: Gymnastics injuries. *Orthop Clin North Am* 1980; 11:717–726.
6. Howell DW: Musculoskeletal profile and incidence of musculoskeletal injuries in light weight women rowers. *Am J Sports Med* 1984; 12(4):278–282.
7. Jackson CP, Brown MD: Analysis of current approaches and a practical guide to prescription of exercise. *Clin Orthop* 1983; 179:46–54.
8. Jackson CP, Brown MD: Is there a role for exercise in the treatment of patients with low back pain? *Clin Orthop* 1983; 179:39–45.
9. Jackson DW, Wiltse LL, Cirincione RJ: Spondylolysis in female gymnasts. *Clin Orthop* 1976; 117:68–73.
10. Kendall PH, Jenkins JS: Exercise for backache: A double-blind controlled trial. *Physiotherapy* 1968; 54:154.
11. Kulund DN: The torso, hip and thigh, in Kulund DN (ed): *The Injured Athlete.* Philadelphia, JB Lippincott Co, 1982, pp 343–350.
12. Lorenz M, McCulloch J: Chemonucleolysis for herniated nucleus pulposus in adolescents. *J Bone Joint Surg Am* 1985; 67:1402–1404.

13. Micheli LJ, Hall JE, Miller ME: Use of modified Boston brace for back injuries in athletes. *Am J Sports Med* 1980; 8(5):351–356.
14. Micheli LJ: Use of modified Boston Brace System (B.O.B.) for back pain: Clinical indications, in *B.O.B.: The Boston Overlap Brace Manual.* Avon, Mass, O&P Systems Inc, 1985.
15. Nachemson AL, Lindh M: Measurement of abdominal and back strength with and without low back pain. *Scand J Rehabil Med* 1969; 1:160.
16. Nachemson A: Work for all. *Clin Orthop* 1983; 179:77–85.
17. O'Donaghue DH: Injuries of the spine, in O'Donaghue DH (ed): *Treatment of Injuries to Athletes.* Philadelphia, WB Saunders Co, 1984, pp 362–406.
18. Pederson OF, Peterson R, Staffedt ES: Back pain and isometric back muscle strength of workers in a Danish factory. *Scand J Rehabil Med* 1975; 7:125.
19. Winter RB: The spine, in Lovell WW, Winter RB (eds): *Pediatric Orthopedics.* Philadelphia, JB Lippincott Co, 1978, pp 680–681.

CHAPTER 8

The Shoulder

The shoulder consists of several joints that effect a complex series of motions and interactions between the upper extremity and trunk.

The three joints that comprise the shoulder are the glenohumeral, the acromioclavicular, and the sternoclavicular. The glenohumeral joint is the most frequently injured joint, as a result of both trauma and overuse. The acromioclavicular joint is frequently injured as result of trauma sustained in football or ice hockey.

In addition to acute and chronic pain, limited range of motion is a major sequela of shoulder injuries. These injuries can be placed into several categories: acute trauma, overuse injuries, and injuries due to degenerative changes. In overuse injuries, the pain is insidious and persistent. The "coracoacromial impingement syndrome" is the prototype. The rotator cuff rupture in the middle-aged athlete is an example of injury due to degenerative changes in the tendinous structures.

As with all athletic injuries, an accurate and detailed history is the key to making the proper diagnosis. In the shoulder region, the importance of this is magnified because of the complex anatomy and biomechanics associated with athletic activity.

THE STERNOCLAVICULAR JOINT

The sternoclavicular joint is made up of the sternum and the clavicle, which are connected by the sternoclavicular and costoclavicular ligaments. The former serves to join the clavicle to the sternum, while the latter prevents elevation of the proximal clavicle. A fibrocartilaginous disk permits the joint to move in several directions.[13]

INJURY: SPRAINS

This joint is subject to sprain, both mild and severe, and to dislocation, although these injuries are rare. First-degree sprains involve stretching of the costoclavicular ligament without resulting instability. A second-degree sprain of the sternoclavicular and costoclavicular ligaments results in laxity and instability of the sternoclavicular joint. A third-degree sprain, which involves dislocation or subluxation, occurs when both ligaments are severely damaged. Dislocation or subluxation can occur in the anterior or posterior direction.

INJURY: DISLOCATIONS

Anterior dislocation results in upward and forward displacement of the medial end of the clavicle.[3] It is characterized by swelling, grating, clicking, and popping with arm elevation and shoulder rotation, and a visible prominence.[8]

Retrosternal or posterior dislocation of the clavicle can be a life-threatening injury if the clavicle impinges upon the great vessels of the neck.[8] Symptoms include a snorting type of breathing, dysphagia, and neurovascular problems. Immediate reduction is necessary.

Mild sprains can be treated with cold, compression, medication (local injections and/or oral analgesics), and sling immobilization. A Velpeau's sling can be applied for seven to ten days, along with a felt or foam pad.

In order to allow damaged ligaments to heal, the shoulder should be put at rest by limiting painful activity.

Problem: Limited Motion and Loss of Strength
REHABILITATION

Following the immobilization period it is important to regain any motion that may have been lost. *Program 1*, the shoulder rehabilitation program, as described in the section on glenohumeral subluxations and dislocations is recommended. This program includes Codman-type pendulum exercises, shoulder abduction, and shoulder flexion range-of-motion exercises. Refer to this section for illustrations and complete descriptions. Progression can be made to strengthening exercises including *program 2*, the isotonic program, described in the section on glenohumeral injuries, and *program 5*, the Nautilus exercises, described at the end of this chapter.

INJURY: CLAVICULAR SHAFT FRACTURES

Clavicular fractures account for 5% to 10% of all fractures occurring in children.[3] Most fractures to this area occur in the middle or outer third of the clavicle.[13] The mechanism of injury can include a direct blow to the front of the shoulder, or a fall on the shoulder or an outstretched arm.[3, 8] Clinical findings include a drooping shoulder, tenderness directly over the shaft, a palpable deformity, pain, and crepitus with motion.

While contusions can be treated with cryotherapy, and the use of proper padding for return to activity, immobilization will be required for fractures. Figure-of-eight clavicular splints, with foam rubber padding over the fracture site, can be used for reduction and immobilization. This is followed by the use of a sling for two to three weeks.[3] The immobilization period should be consistent with adequate bone healing.

Problem: Loss of Motion and Strength

REHABILITATION

The predominant problem following immobilization for fractures is the limitation of range of motion. *Program 1*, the shoulder rehabilitation program, should be instituted as early as possible after healing. In addition, strengthening exercise are necessary. Progression can be made to isotonic strengthening exercises, *program 2*, and Nautilus, *program 5*.

ACROMIOCLAVICULAR JOINT

The acromioclavicular joint consists of the articulation of the clavicle to the anteromedial aspect of the acromion by the acromioclavicular ligament, which provides stability between the clavicle and the scapula. The coracoclavicular ligaments prevent upward displacement of the clavicle.[13]

INJURY: SPRAINS

The mechanism of injury is usually a downward blow against the outer end of the shoulder, which drives the acromion down, and the clavicle up. Falling on an outstretched arm or a flexed elbow can also cause this type of injury. Sprains of the acromioclavicular joint are commonly referred to as "shoulder separations."

First-degree sprains, or mild sprains, are slight tears of the acromioclavicular or coracoclavicular ligaments, and they are characterized by localized pain at the acromioclavicular joint and pain with overhead movement. There is no demonstrable instability on clinical examination or roentgenogram.

Moderate sprains, or second-degree sprains, involve more extensive damage to the ligaments. Usually there is a complete tear of the acromioclavicular ligament, and a partial tear of the coracoclavicular ligament. Symptoms include swelling, a notable prominence at the joint, a movable distal clavicle, pain with any active overhead movement, and tenderness at the joint. This is associated with subluxation of the joint.

Third-degree sprains are severe, and involve complete tearing of both the acromioclavicular and coracoclavicular ligaments. In the third-degree injury there is more swelling and tenderness than in the less severe types. There is pain with manipulation, and an upward riding at the outer end of the clavicle. These injuries are usually caused by a direct blow to the outer edge of the shoulder on an outstretched arm. There is dislocation with complete separation.[13]

Conservative treatment consisting of cryotherapy and immobilization with a Kenny Howard sling can be used for all three kinds of sprains. First-degree sprains may not require immobilization, but the use of protective padding for return to activity is recommended. The Kenny Howard sling forces the humerus up and the clavicle down, thereby relieving the dislocation and allowing the ligamentous structures to heal in an anatomical position. The sling is worn 24 hours a day for four to six weeks. While immobilization is advocated for second-degree sprains, its use in treating third-degree sprains is controversial. Internal fixation is advocated by many, via pin, screw, or internal tape fixation.

Problem: Loss of Motion and Strength

REHABILITATION

Following immobilization in the Kenny Howard sling, range of motion will be limited. *Program 1*, the shoulder rehabilitation program described in the section on glenohumeral subluxations and dislocations, can be followed.

Strengthening

Strengthening should include a program that exercises all the muscle groups of the shoulder girdle and upper arm. *Program 2*, the isotonic shoulder program is described in the section on glenohumeral subluxation and dislocations. In the early phases of strengthening the arm should not be raised above a level parallel to the floor. It is important that exercises be performed only within the pain-free range of motion.

INJURY: CHRONIC LESIONS OF THE ACROMIOCLAVICULAR JOINT

Repeated minor strains of the capsular ligament of the acromioclavicular joint can lead to the development of chronic inflammatory lesions and osteoarthritis in the joint. Arthritic changes can occur with heavy repetitive use of the joint that often occurs in contact sports and with weightlifting.[13] Symptoms include pain with shoulder movement, especially abduction and flexion above 90 degrees, pain while sleeping on the affected side, tenderness over the acromioclavicular joint, and pain with upward compression and downward pull on the joint.[3]

Rest, application of ice, and the injection of a long-acting local anesthetic and corticosteroid preparation are usually effective in controlling symptoms.[3, 13] Surgery may be necessary if conservative treatment is not effective. Resectioning of 1 or 2 cm of the distal end of the clavicle is usually the surgery of choice. Full return to activity following complete rehabilitation is usually possible.[13]

REHABILITATION

Care must be taken in prescribing vigorous motion and weight-training exercises in cases in which degenerative changes are a factor.

GLENOHUMERAL JOINT/ROTATOR CUFF

The glenohumeral joint consists of the head of the humerus, which rests in the glenoid fossa, and the muscle tendons, which make up the rotator cuff and function as stabilizers. The supraspinatus, infraspinatus, and teres minor attach to the greater tuberosity, and the subscapularis to the lesser tuberosity.

INJURY: GLENOHUMERAL SUBLUXATION

Anterior-inferior subluxation is a common shoulder injury.[13] It can occur when there is a disruption of the glenohumeral ligaments, cartilaginous labrum, and/ or bony glenoid. Subluxation of the humeral head anteriorly, and over the rim of the glenoid can occur when such deficiencies exist.[13] The symptoms include a feeling of slipping with overhead activity, muscle spasm, and pain on abduction/external rotation. Often, the patient reports that there is a feeling that the shoulder can dislocate or has dislocated.[13]

Recurrent posterior glenohumeral subluxation is characterized by pain with adduction and forward flexion, and limited external rotation. These posterior injuries can be acute, recurrent, or permanent. Some authors claim that posterior dislocations are subluxations that develop over time.[12]

INJURY: GLENOHUMERAL DISLOCATION

Anterior dislocation is characterized by pain, disability, and pain with movement. Anterior-inferior dislocation is a common injury among young athletes.[13] Forcing the arm into complete abduction can result in inferior dislocation.

Recurrent dislocations may be broken into several categories. The most common is recurrent anterior dislocation. It can be the result of either repeated traumatic dislocation in normal shoulders, or of repeated dislocation due to congenital deviation around the glenohumeral joint.[13] There is reported to be a 80% recurrence rate in individuals younger than 40 years. The second category for recurrent dislocations is recurrent posterior dislocations.

The traditional method for managing shoulder dislocations consisted of immobilization for three to six weeks, with the shoulder in adduction and internal rotation. Based on a study comparing those immobilized to those not immobilized, Henry and Genung[6] concluded that (1) the prognosis of recurrent dislocation was not affected significantly by immobilization; (2) the amount of time between injury and recurrence was not related to immobilization or the length of immobilization; (3) there is a high recurrence rate for this injury among high school students; and (4) immobilization for three to six weeks does not alter the recurrence rate.[6]

Problem: Loss of Motion and Strength

REHABILITATION

Program 1: Shoulder Rehabilitation Program

The following program can be followed to improve range of motion, which is often limited after immobilization.

Range-Of-Motion Exercises.—The Codman exercises are effective in improving range of motion, which decreases following muscular injury or a lengthy period of immobilization. They should be performed as follows:

1. Bend forward at the waist, so that the upper body is at a 45 to 90 degree angle to the hips. Hold onto a chair or table with the opposite hand for balance.
2. Swing the arm from side to side, drawing a horizontal line, and repeat for two minutes (Fig 8–1,A).
3. With the body in the same position, swing the arm backward and forward, drawing a vertical line, and repeat for two minutes (Fig 8–1,B).
4. With the injured arm, draw a circle with a 6- to 18-in. diameter, in the clockwise direction (Fig 8–1,C) for 2 minutes.
5. Repeat the exercise in Step 4, this time drawing a circle in the counterclockwise position for 2 minutes.

Shoulder Abduction (to be done for 10 minutes).—Follow the steps given below.

1. Begin by lying supine on the floor, arm fully extended against the body.
2. Abduct the arm away from the body, by "walking" it with the fingers.
3. Abduct it to the point at which a gentle stretch is felt; hold it for 10 seconds (Fig 8–2,A).
4. Continue to abduct the arm until another stretch position is reached, and again hold it for 10 seconds.
5. Continue in this manner until the arm is extended 90 degrees from the body (Fig 8–2,B).
6. Progression to greater range of motion can be made approximately two weeks after reaching 90 degrees of extension (Fig 8–2,C).

Shoulder Flexion.—Follow the steps given below.

1. Stand with arm at side, elbow extended, palm against the thigh.
2. Raise the arm in front of the body until it is parallel to the floor.
3. Hold this position for 6 seconds.
4. Return arm to side; rest for 2 seconds.
5. Repeat 8–12 times (Figs 8–3,A and B demonstrate flexion using a dumbbell weight).

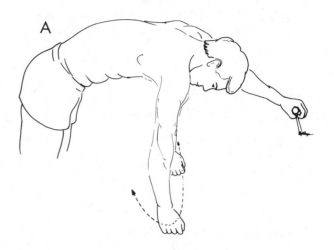

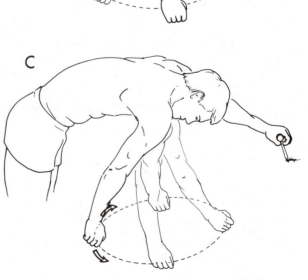

FIG 8–1.
A, the Codman pendulum horizontal arm swing exercise. Bend forward at the waist so that the body is at a 45 to 90 degree angle to the hips, and hold onto a table or chair for support. Draw a horizontal line by swinging the injured arm from side to side. **B,** the Codman pendulum vertical arm swing exercise. Bend forward at the waist so that the body is at a 45 to 90 degree angle to the hips, and hold onto the back of a chair for support. Draw a vertical line by swinging the injured arm back and forth. **C,** the Codman pendulum arm circle exercise. Bend foward at waist so that the body is at a 45 to 90 degree angle to the hips, and hold onto the back of a chair for support. Draw a circle with a 6- to 8-in. diameter in the clockwise direction with the injured arm. Repeat in the counterclockwise position as well.

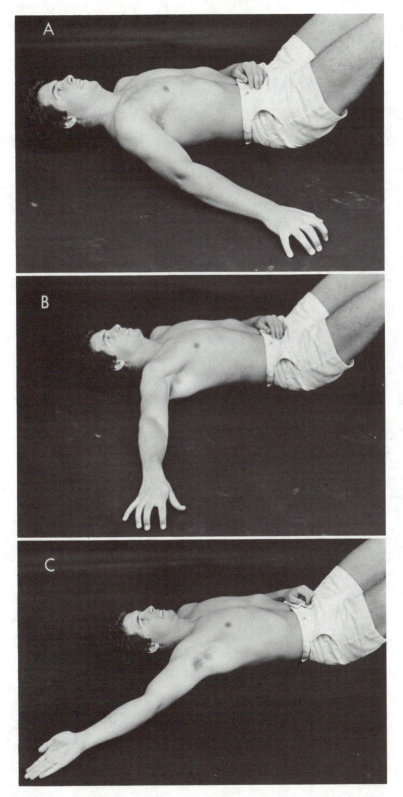

FIG 8–2.
Range of motion. **A,** abduction to 45 degrees. Lie supine on the floor with the arm extended next to the body. Begin to abduct the arm, walking with the fingers along the floor, until the arm is at a 45 degree angle. **B,** abduction to 90 degrees. **C,** abduction to 120 degrees.

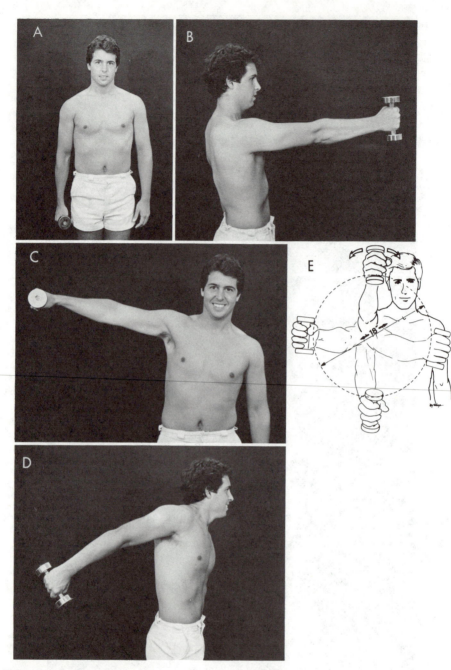

FIG 8–3.

Isotonic exercises. **A,** the starting position for the three isotonic exercises. In the standing position, hold a dumbbell in the hand of the affected arm, keeping the arm by the side and fully extended. **B,** the shoulder flexion exercise. Raise the arm forward until it is parallel with the floor. Hold this position for 2 seconds. Lower and repeat. **C,** the shoulder abduction exercise. Starting as in **A,** raise the arm from the side until it is parallel with the floor. Hold this position for 2 seconds. **D,** the shoulder extension exercise. Starting from position **A,** raise the arm backward as far as possible without bending at the waist or leaning forward. Hold this position for 2 seconds. Lower and repeat. **E,** the shoulder circle exercise with 18-in. diameter. Hold a dumbbell in hand and extend the arm in front of the body until it is parallel with the floor. Make 18-in. diameter circles, both clockwise and counterclockwise.

Shoulder Abduction.—Follow the steps given below.

1. Stand with the arm at the side, elbow extended, palm against the thigh (see Fig 8–3,A).
2. Abduct the arm from the side of the body until it is parallel to the floor.
3. Hold this position for 6 seconds.
4. Lower the arm; rest for 2 seconds.
5. Repeat 8–12 times (Fig 8–3,C demonstrates abduction using a dumbbell weight).
6. Apply ice to the shoulder for 20 minutes immediately after completing the last exercise.
   This program should be done 2 times per day.

Strength Training

Once range of motion has improved, progression can be made to strengthening exercises as described in *program 2*, the isotonic exercise program. The internal rotator muscles, namely, the subscapularis, should be given priority in strength training; therefore, the internal rotation exercises described should be emphasized.

Program 2: Isotonic Program

This program is performed with dumbbell weights.

Shoulder Flexion (supraspinatus, infraspinatus, teres minor, subscapularis).—Follow the steps given below.

1. Stand with the arm at the side, and the elbow fully extended (see Fig 8–3, A).
2. Raise the arm up in front of the body until it is parallel with the floor (see Fig 8–3, B).
3. Hold this position for 1 to 2 seconds.
4. Slowly return the arm to the starting position.

Shoulder Abduction (deltoid, supraspinatous).—Follow the steps given below.

1. Stand with the arm at the side, and the elbow fully extended (see Fig 8–3,A).
2. Abduct the arm away from the side of the body until it is parallel with the floor (Fig 8–3,C).
3. Hold this position for 1 to 2 seconds.
4. Slowly return to starting position.

Shoulder Extension (deltoid, teres minor).—Follow the steps given below.

1. Stand with the arm at the side, and the elbow fully extended (see Fig 8–3,A).

2. Extend the arm straight back as far as possible without bending at the waist (Fig 8–3,D).
3. Hold this position for 1 to 2 seconds.
4. Slowly return to the starting position.

Shoulder Circles.—Follow the steps given below.

1. Stand with the arm at the side and the elbow fully extended (see Fig 8–3,A).
2. Extend the arm in front of the body until it is parallel with the floor.
3. Make an 18-in. diameter circle in the clockwise position.
4. Make an 18-in. diameter circle in the counterclockwise direction (Fig 8–3,E).

Internal Rotation.—Follow the steps given below.

1. Stand with upper arms against the side of the chest; bend elbows to 90 degrees, palms up.
2. Grasp a broomstick with hands 18 in. apart (Fig 8–4,A).
3. Try to push hands together for 10 seconds, but do not allow the hands to slip along the stick.
4. Repeat with the hands 12 in. apart.
5. Repeat with the hands 6 in. apart.

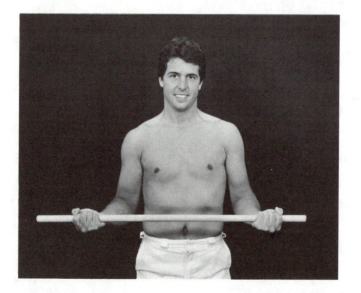

FIG 8–4.
Internal and external rotation isometrics with the broomstick. For internal rotation: While standing, and with the upper arm against the side, flex the elbows to 90 degrees, and with the palms up, grasp the broomstick. Begin with the hands 18 in. apart, and keeping the hands in one place as shown, try to push them toward each other. Exert pressure for 6 seconds. Relax, then repeat. Repeat this series with the hands 12 in. apart and 6 in. apart. For external rotation: Begin as with internal rotation, except begin with the hands 6 in. apart. Try to pull the hands apart, but do not allow them to slip along the broomstick handle. Pull for 6 seconds; relax and repeat. Repeat the series with the hands 12 and 18 in. apart.

External Rotation.—Follow the steps given below.
Phase 1.—

1. Stand with upper arms against the side of the chest; bend elbows to 90 degrees, palms up.
2. Grasp a broomstick, hands should be 6 in. apart.
3. Try to pull hands apart for 10 seconds, do not allow hands to slip.
4. Repeat with hands 12 in. apart.
5. Repeat with hands 18 in. apart (see Fig 8–4,A).

Phase 2.—To work external rotation of the right shoulder, apply pressure to the end of the broomstick with the left hand, moving the right shoulder into external rotation (Figs 8–5,A and B).

The following program should be done:
1. Shoulder flexion—ten repetitions.
2. Shoulder abduction—ten repetitions.
3. Shoulder extension—ten repetitions.
4. Shoulder circles—clockwise—ten repetitions.
5. Shoulder circles—counterclockwise—ten repetitions.
Repeat this sequence two or more times for a total of three sets. Then:
1. Shoulder external rotation—ten repetitions.
2. Shoulder internal rotation—ten repetitions.
Apply ice to the shoulder for 20 minutes.
It is important to note that good form must always be maintained in order to achieve the full benefit of these exercises. Try to increase the amount of weight lifted by 2½ lb every 7 to 14 days.
It has been observed that while these treatments are appropriate, the intended results—namely, improvements in flexibility and muscular endurance and the return to normal range of motion—are not achieved through these exercises alone. Strengthening exercises that are designed to specifically rehabilitate the rotator cuff muscles are often times not prescribed or are performed incorrectly.[4]

INJURY: ROTATOR CUFF LESIONS

The rotator cuff muscles include the supraspinatus, infraspinatus, teres minor, and subscapularis. These join together to form the tendon cuff that inserts at the anatomic head of the humerus.[18] The synergistic contraction of the short rotators and the deltoid produces the movement of abduction or flexion. The supraspinatus is referred to by Codman as the "initiator of abduction." Impingement had been defined by Neer, cited by Hawkins and Kennedy,[5] as the impingement of the anterior portion of the acromion with its attached coracoacromial ligament on the critical area of the rotator cuff and biceps tendon.[18] Subluxation, dislocation of the glenohumeral joint, fracture of the greater tuberosity, or degeneration of cuff tissue can cause rotator cuff tears. Also, poor blood supply to this area is cited as reason for susceptibility of this area to injury.[10, 18]

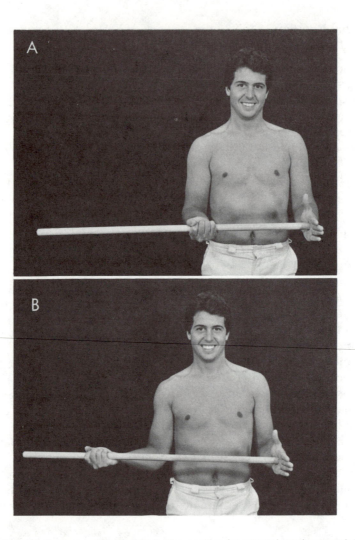

FIG 8–5.
External rotation with the broomstick. **A,** the starting position for external rotation stretch for the right shoulder using the broomstick. Flex the right elbow to 90 degrees and hold the broomstick in the right hand, palm facing up. Place the left hand at the end of the broomstick. **B,** External rotation of the right shoulder using the broomstick. From the position in **A,** move the broomstick to the right by applying pressure to the end with the left hand. Hold the stretching position for 6 seconds. Relax and repeat. Repeat the exercise for the opposite shoulder.

Injuries to the biceps tendon will be discussed separately later, as will frozen shoulder, which also accompanies cuff tears.[19]

There are two categories of cuff tears, partial and complete. Partial tears are most common[8] and are characterized by pain during overhead motions, crepitus and clicking, weakness of the abductors,[8] and the necessary signs of adhesive capsulitis and tendinitis.[3, 17] Both injuries result in pain, cuff tenderness, painful and limited range of motion, limited passive rotation, pain on resisted movement, and with attempted active abduction or external rotation.[8] Difficulty in initiating abduction is also sign of supraspinatus tear as in the "drop arm sign" or failure to maintain a position of 90 degrees of abduction when positioned passively by the examiner.[19] In individuals over 40 years old, rotator cuff tears are often a cause of shoulder dysfunction and shoulder pain.[9] Injury to the supraspinatus tendon is characterized by a "tearing" or "snap," a short, pain-free interval, recurring pain for several days, and tenderness.[17] Chronic injuries are characterized by continued soreness and progressive stiffness. Weakness of abduction will still be present. Massive tears are indicated by inability to abduct.[19]

Conservative treatment should be tried for a reasonable amount of time in the case of rotator cuff tears.[19] The great majority of patients with rotator cuff tears will recover sufficiently without surgery. Depolonas, cited by Wolfgang,[19] outlines five advantages for nonsurgical treatment that have been voiced in the past: (1) most patients recover without surgery; (2) delayed repairs do as well as immediate ones; nothing is lost by waiting; (3) degenerated tendon heals poorly, and resection of the scarred edges creates tension of the sutured area; (4) surgery often does not restore normal function; and (5) surgical complications are frequent, including weakness, detachment of the deltoid repair, undesirable scars, and residual impingement.[19] This approach would involve a sling as the simplest method of immobilization and the use of medication (analgesics, anti-inflammatory agents).[19]

Problem: Limited Range of Motion

Immobilization for cuff tears will result in limited range of motion. Exercises that will restore this lost motion are described following the section on adhesive capsulitis.

Problem: Limited Strength

Once range of motion has been regained, individuals can perform strengthening exercises specifically for injuries to the rotator cuff. These also follow the stretching section after adhesive capsulitis section.

INJURY: FROZEN SHOULDER/ADHESIVE CAPSULITIS

Adhesive capsulitis is characterized by inflammatory edema and contracture of fibrous tissue about the glenohumeral joint.[17] Range of motion of the joint should be assessed. Abduction and external humeral rotation characteristically become limited. The motion of abduction and rotation causes soreness that increases gradually and eventually develops into constant pain and disability. However, it does not interfere with sleep. The chronic stage sees the subsiding of pain and disability with varying degrees of limited motion remaining. When this problem goes untreated, an immobile, or frozen, shoulder results.[17]

The acute stage can be treated with local cooling to relieve pain, inflammation, and muscle spasm. The subacute stage can be treated with superficial heating; the increased blood flow prevents the destruction of collagen tissue.[17] Nonnarcotic analgesics can be administered.[9] See Chapter 12 for further details on the use of this medication. The subacute and chronic stages should be treated with intensive range of motion program.

Rehabilitation Exercises

The exercise period should consist of heating the shoulder area, forward flexion movement with assistance from the other arm, external rotation movement with the aid of a broomstick handle, as well as shoulder extension and internal rotation movements. Records of changes in range of motion in these directions are kept. Gains are said to be slow but progressive. Ten to 15 degrees of forward flexion are usually gained per month. Exercises should be continued even after full function has been regained.[9]

Stretching Exercises: Upper Extremity

In addition to range of motion exercises, such as the Codman exercises, and abduction exercises, as described in *program 1*, stretching is also important. In recreational or competitive sports, a warm-up program is designed to decrease the risk of potential injury or reinjury to the participants. A sound warm-up routine, including stretching exercises, will enhance the safety of the activity.

The stretching exercises presented concentrate on flexibility work for the upper extremity. Basic considerations for performing the exercises are as follows: (1) do not force a stretch by bouncing; (2) move the limb segment through its range of motion approaching the point of stretch; hold at this point for approximately 6 to 10 seconds; (3) if the goal is to maintain flexibility, three repetitions of each exercise will suffice. However to gain flexibility, six to ten repetitions should be completed; and (4) stretching exercises should be done before and after an activity session.

Program 3: Stretching and Range of Motion

The following stretching exercises are specifically for rotator cuff injuries, and can follow program 1, described earlier in the chapter.

Shoulder and Upper Arm Stretch.—Gently pull the arm across the back of the head. Reverse direction to feel stretch in opposite arm.

Horizontal Adductor Stretch.—With the elbow flexed to 60 degrees, and the arm abducted to 90 degrees, horizontally adduct the arm by using pressure with the opposite hand (Fig 8–6).

Overhead Stretch.—Place the hands on the broomstick as shown in Figure 8–7,A. With the arms extended, raise overhead until a stretch is felt.

Shoulder and Trunk Stretch.—Grasp a broomstick handle as shown in Figure 8–7,A. Raise arms overhead and stretch upward. Maintain this position

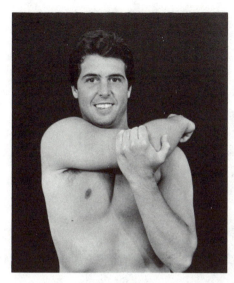

FIG 8–6.
Horizontal adduction. The stretching position for horizontal adduction. Abduct the arm to 90 degrees, and then horizontally adduct it, with the elbow flexed to about 60 degrees. Gently apply pressure with the opposite hand to further assist horizontal adduction. This exercise can be repeated for the opposite arm.

for 6 seconds and slowly lean to the side to involve trunk muscles. Repeat in the opposite direction (Fig 8–7,B).

Internal and External Rotator Stretch.—Follow directions given below.

Internal rotation.—Hold a broomstick behind the back as shown in Figure 8–8,A. Gently pull downward on the broomstick with the left hand until a stretch is felt in the right arm. Hold for 6 to 8 seconds. Repeat this exercise for the left arm by reversing the position.

External rotation.—Hold a broomstick behind the back as shown in Figure 8–8,B. Gently pull up on the broomstick with the left hand and feel the stretch in the right shoulder. Hold for 6 to 8 seconds. This exercise can be repeated for the opposite shoulder by reversing the position of the arms.

Horizontal Abductor Stretch (3-s Technique).—With the arms extended behind, a partner provides resistance while the patient attempts to pull forward. The 3-s technique for stretching is explained in the section on swimmer's shoulder.

Program 4: Rotator Cuff Strengthening

Abduction Diagonal Pattern (for supraspinatus).—Follow the instructions given below.

Position.—Arm extended along the side of the body with the hand turned inward.

Action.—Abduct the arm in a diagonal pattern through 45 degrees of motion; if there is no difficulty through limited range of motion, motion can be increased through 90 degrees or until the arm is parallel to the floor (Fig 8–9).

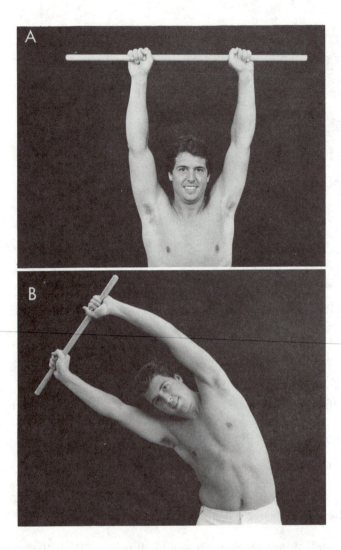

FIG 8–7.
A, the starting position for the lateral bending stretching exercise. Hold a broomstick overhead, keeping the hands shoulder-distance apart and the arms straight. Stretch upward and hold for 6 seconds. **B,** the stretching position for the lateral bend exercise. Slowly lean to the right and feel the stretch in the trunk and left side. Repeat this exercise in the opposite direction.

Shoulder External Rotation (To strengthen the infraspinatus, teres minor, and subscapularis).—Follow the instructions given below.

Position.—Lying on the unaffected side, place the upper arm of the affected shoulder against the side of the upper body; bend the elbow and place the hand on the abdomen (Fig 8–10,A).

Action.—Externally rotate, raising the weight upward, hold for 2 seconds, lower and repeat (Fig 8–10,B).

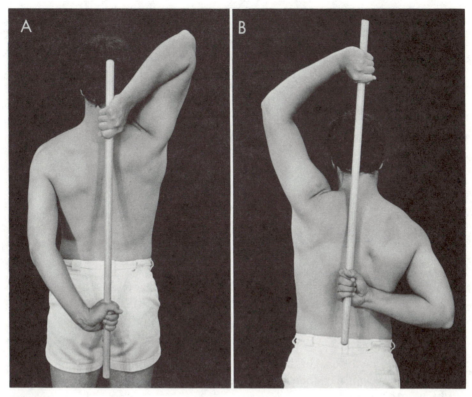

FIG 8–8.
Internal/external rotation stretching—broomstick. **A,** internal rotation stretching exercise for the right shoulder. Hold a broomstick behind the back as shown. Gently pull down on the broomstick with the left hand and feel the stretch in the right arm. Repeat this exercise for the left arm by reversing the position of the arms. **B,** external rotation stretching exercise for the right shoulder. Hold a broomstick behind the back as shown. Gently pull up on the broomstick with the left hand and feel the stretch in the right shoulder. This exercise can be repeated for the opposite shoulder by reversing the position of the arms.

Shoulder Internal Rotation.—Follow the instructions given below.

Position.—Lying on the affected side, tuck the upper arm in against the chest, and bend the elbow to 90 degrees (Fig 8–11,A).

Action.—Internally rotate, bringing the arm upward toward the stomach; hold for 2 seconds, lower and repeat (Fig 8–11,B).

Frequency

Exercises should be performed once a day, Monday through Friday, at the onset.

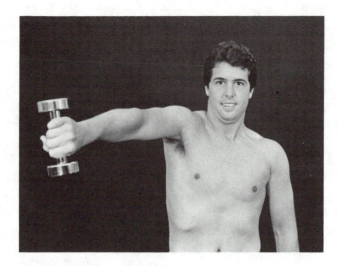

FIG 8–9.
Rotator cuff strengthening: diagonal abduction. The diagonal abduction exercise using the dumbbell weight. Begin standing, with the hand and arm hanging to the side. Internally rotate the arm and abduct it until it is parallel with the floor. Hold the position shown for 1 to 2 seconds; relax and repeat. If range of motion in the arm is limited, abduct to 90 degrees as shown here.

Resistance

Begin with a light weight, 2 to 3 lb. If no increased soreness develops in the shoulder, the weight can then be increased to 2 to 3 lb. The target weight will not be more than 10 lb.

Sets/Repetitions

Perform three sets of ten repetitions. One set of ten repetitions should be done of each exercise. The sequence should then be completed two more times for a total of three sets.

Stretching exercises should be completed before and after each exercise session. After exercising, ice should be applied for 20 minutes.

Cryotherapy

When active range of motion is used, local cooling is recommended to decrease inflammation and pain during the acute stage.[17]

Strength Training: Nautilus and Cybex

Progression can be made from the rotator cuff strengthening exercise program to Nautilus (see program 5). Again, it is important that exercises be performed only within the pain-free range of motion. As with Nautilus equipment, the Cybex is an excellent tool for rehabilitating the shoulder. Its value is found in strengthening and increasing muscular endurance. In addition, it is ideal for performing proprioceptive neuromuscular patterning following injury and surgery. A variety of muscle groups and movements can be exercised.

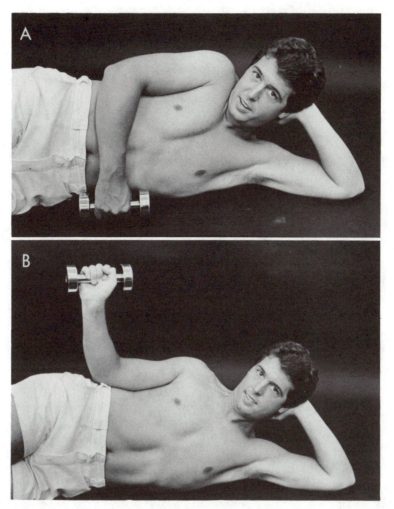

FIG 8–10.
A, the starting position for external rotation strengthening exercise. Lie on the unaffected side, place the upper arm against the side of the trunk, and internally rotate the arm until the hand rests on the stomach. **B,** the arm in the fully externally rotated position. From position **A,** keep the upper arm against the body; raise the weight, directing the back of the hand to the wall behind. Hold this position for 2 seconds. Lower to position **A.** Repeat for 3 sets of 10 repetitions.

Surgical Treatment

There is disagreement over whether painful rotator cuff tears should be treated surgically. Indication for surgery was the failure of conservative treatment following three months of its administration. Post et al. report on the repair of 59 shoulders in 55 patients. The amount of pain experienced and the degree of function present were used as indicators for success or failure of surgery. Post concluded that early surgical repair with partial anterior acromionectomy is recommended for rotator cuff tears. Early repair produced more success than late repair in his particular population.[14]

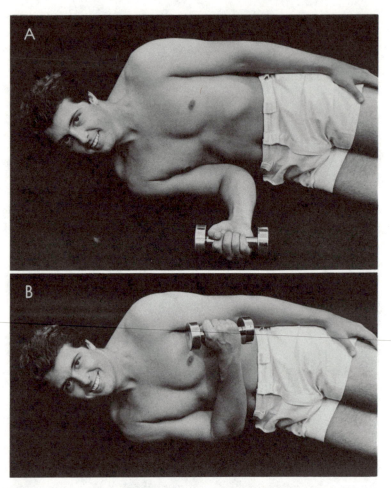

FIG 8–11.
Rotator cuff strengthening—internal/external rotation. **A,** the starting position for the internal rotation strengthening exercise. Lie on the affected side; tuck the upper arm of the injured shoulder against the chest and flex the elbow to 90 degrees. **B,** the arm in the fully internally rotated position. Keeping the upper arm tucked against the chest; raise the weight by rotating it toward the abdomen. Hold for 2 seconds and return to position **A.** Repeat for 3 sets of 10 repetitions.

Problem: Loss of Motion and Strength

REHABILITATION

Follow the same sequence as described for nonsurgical rehabilitation—namely, rehabilitation *Programs 1, 3, 4, and 5.* Again, emphasis is on improving range of motion and strength.

INJURY: ROTATOR CUFF TENDINITIS

Calcific Tendinitis

The pain characterizing this form of tendinitis is sharp, localized, and severe.[9] Additional symptoms include a disruption of shoulder function, localized tenderness with palpation of the injured portion of the cuff, and increase in discomfort with active or passive stretch of the affected tendon. Among the tendons that may be involved are the supraspinatus, the infraspinatus, subscapularis, biceps, and, occasionally, the teres minor.[9] Relief can be attained through rest and administration of analgesics and anti-inflammatory agents. Surgical resection of the calcium deposit may be required for chronic or recurrent cases.

REHABILITATION

Stretching Exercises: Upper Extremity

The stretching exercises described under the section on the rehabilitation of rotator cuff lesions and adhesive capsulitis (program 3) should be a part of the treatment of calcific tendinitis. Refer to this section for descriptions and illustrations.

INJURY: BICIPITAL TENOSYNOVITIS, BICIPITAL TENDINITIS, STRAIN OF THE LONG HEAD OF THE BICEPS

Anterior shoulder pain may be due to impingement, subluxation, or strain of the tendon of the long head of the biceps. The anatomical positioning of the tendon in the intertubercle groove of the humerus predisposes it to chronic irritation.[1] Bicipital tenosynovitis and tendinitis are aggravated by repetitive glenohumeral motion that involves internal rotation and circumduction or extension of the humerus.

INJURY: SUBLUXATION OF THE BICEPS TENDON

Irritation of the biceps tendon as it subluxes out of the bicipital groove causes pain. Abduction to 90 degrees with forced internal or external rotation may produce the symptom. Anterior shoulder pain, popping, cracking, and locking sensations are also felt at times.[8]

INJURY: BICIPITAL TENDINITIS

This injury also results in tenderness over the biceps groove. It can be diagnosed with the Yergason test; starting with the elbow flexed at a 90 degree angle and the palm of the hand facing down, the patient supinates his forearm against resistance supplied by the examiner. Pain in the bicipital groove may indicate bicipital tendinitis.[3] Irritation and inflammation of the insertion of the short head of the biceps into the choracoid process is a frequent problem in gymnasts, and if not treated, it can become chronic.[3, 8]

INJURY: BICEPS TENDON RUPTURES

When the biceps tendon ruptures, a bulging biceps muscle results along with a palpable defect. Ruptures can occur in three different locations: (1) where the tendon originates in the supraglenoid fossa, (2) in the bicipital groove, or (3) at the musculotendinous juncture in the upper arm.[3] The pain may be intense after an acute rupture, or mild and recurrent and accompanied by stiffness.[3]

The following treatment program can be used for proximal biceps problems: surgical neglect, application of ice, the administration of oral anti-inflammatory agents, and rest followed by vigorous rehabilitation. Surgical repair is indicated for distal tendinous ruptures.

REHABILITATION

The range of motion and stretching exercises described in the section on rotator cuff *(program 3)* can be followed, and strengthening exercises, including shoulder rehabilitation *program 2* and elbow flexion (see Chapter 10), are recommended.

INJURY: BURSITIS

Acute subacromial, chronic subacromial, and subscapularis bursitis are three problems that can occur in the shoulder region.[8, 13] Gordon[3] explains that what is usually referred to as bursitis is characterized by pain that originates in the subacromial region, and is caused by abduction and external rotation. He states that the injury actually involves the musculotendinous cuff and the biceps tendon and sheath, and not just the bursa. When the arm is abducted laterally through the range of 70 to 110 degrees, acute pain is experienced. This diminishes as the arm continues upward. Gordon cites the impingement of the inflamed structure beneath the acromion process and the coracoacromial arch as the mechanism behind the pain.[3]

The treatment protocol for bursitis resembles that for impingement syndrome, described in the next section.

INJURY: IMPINGEMENT SYNDROME

Impingement of the shoulder can take several forms and may involve the supraspinatus tendon, biceps tendon, or greater tuberosity. Irritation of these structures by the acromial arch can cause the painful arch syndrome. Two mechanisms can lead to the development of impingement. First, the space under the arch decreases due to an increase in the volumes of the structures within it; this is usually a result of inflammation or edema. Second, the space available for the cuff decreases due to the presence of osteophytes on the inferior and anterior aspects of the acromion.

SUPRASPINATUS TENDINITIS WITH IMPINGEMENT

This is a very common problem. Irritation of the tendon can occur from the repeated pressure on the supraspinatus tendon between the head of the humerus and the acromion. Overuse in the overhead position can produce this condition in young persons, while degenerative changes can contribute to its development in older patients.[5] Degenerative changes in the area of the rotator cuff have been theorized as resulting from the decrease in vascularity that characterizes the area.[5]

Symptoms include gnawing aching pain over the deltoid (which increases with activity), pain at night, minimal tenderness on palpation, pain with abduction (from 60 to 120 degrees[10]) or external rotation against resistance (indicating involvement of the supraspinatus and infraspinatus tendons), discomfort with cross-body adduction or internal rotation. The impingement sign (pain with forced elevation of the humerus against the acromion) will be present. Tendinitis from impingement can be confirmed if a subacromial injection of 5 to 10 ml of lidocaine into the subacromial space relieves pain that comes with impingement.[5] Additional characteristics are point tenderness over the great tuberosity and anterior acromion.[5]

INJURY: BICEPS IMPINGEMENT

This injury results in pain during overhead forward flexion with external rotation. The pain and painful "catching" sensations can be relieved by internal rotation. This distinguishes this injury from supraspinatus impingement, in which the above movement increases pain. This is also characterized by tenderness over the biceps tendon, positive straight arm raising test, consisting of forward flexion of the humerus with the elbow extended, and a positive resisted forearm supination test. Both of these lead to pain in the bicipital groove.[5]

Neer, cited in Hawkins and Kennedy,[5] provides a three-stage classification system for impingement. Edema and hemorrhage comprise stage 1; fibrosis and tendinitis, stage 2; and tendon degeneration, bony changes, and tendon ruptures in persons older than 40 years, stage 3. This injury is not only limited to the acromion and coracoacromial ligament, but may also include the biceps tendon, subacromial bursa, and acromioclavicular joint.[5] The clinical signs and symptoms characterizing the injury include (1) minimal pain with activity, no weakness, no restriction in range of motion; (2) marked reactive tendinitis with significant pain and diminished range of motion; and (3) pain with significant weakness.[5] The diagnosis can be confirmed by performing the "impingement test," which involves elevating the arm forward while in internal rotation, with the scapula fixated manually. Pain will result as the greater tuberosity impinges against the acromion. Relief of this pain with the injection of 10 ml of 1.0% lidocaine beneath the anterior acromion confirms the diagnosis.[5, 8]

Treatment for impingement syndrome can be nonsurgical, including rest without active use of shoulder above the horizontal, anti-inflammatory medication, nonnarcotic analgesics, and application of ice. In chronic cases when pain and weakness persist over months, surgical decompression may be necessary.[16]

Problem: Limited Range of Motion
REHABILITATION

In the case of impingement injuries, range of motion can be limited. Stretching exercises including the ones described in the previous section on rotator cuff lesions and adhesive capsulitis (*program 3*) should be a part of the treatment program for impingement problems. Refer to the above section for descriptions and illustrations of these exercises.

PROBLEM: LOSS OF STRENGTH

Pain-free strengthening of the internal and external rotators is important. *Program 4* outlined for rotator cuff strengthening should be followed carefully. It is important to emphasize that a judicious approach rather than an aggressive approach is essential.

INJURY: SWIMMER'S SHOULDER

Impingement and overuse are responsible for the injury known as swimmer's shoulder. There is a 40% to 60% incidence of painful shoulder among swimmers. The syndrome can be broken down into four phases. The first involves pain only after activity. The second includes pain both during and after activity but normal participation is possible. Phase three is when pain interferes with the normal level of athletic activity, and the fourth is when there is pain during the normal course of the day.[8]

Internal rotation and forward flexion between 60 degrees and 90 degrees with the arm straight overhead, and then pulling the arm down another 30 degrees are the positions that elicit shoulder pain. The typical area of tenderness in swimmer's shoulder is along the coracoacromial ligament and also under the acromion itself.[2] Pain can also occur in the parascapular region and trapezius due to fatigue. Swimmer's shoulder is not generally characterized by significant loss of motion or wasting. Significant swelling, diffuse tenderness, loss of sensation, atrophy, and loss of pulse, are signs indicating a more significant problem.[2]

Rest is a major part of the treatment for swimmer's shoulder.[2] The amount of rest required varies with age. Those under 12 years are advised to rest until complete recovery has occurred. Those over 12 years are not necessarily confined to complete inactivity. They may engage in pain-free swimming or swimming until pain occurs. Additional training alterations may be used, such as training the legs only with the kickboard. For those over 25 years, rest may not be enough because of degenerative processes, precapsulitis, and tendinitis.[2]

Cryotherapy in the form of crushed ice or ice massage can be applied for 10 to 15 minutes, four to five times a day. Alternating ice and heat can be used, but ice is the most important.[2] Medication is helpful in all inflammatory conditions about the shoulder (see Chapter 12 for further details).

Stroke Mechanics

Limiting abduction and internal rotation is the aim of stroke modification. It is during such movement that the impingement of the supraspinatus tendon against the coracoacromial ligament and anterior leading edge of the acromion is most likely to occur. Adduction should also be limited to prevent "wringing out" of the watershed area of hypovascularity in the supraspinatus tendon.[11] The radius of rotation of the arm can be reduced by the high elbow recovery, which also minimizes drag. Front crawl, then, should consist of (1) shortened stroke cadence, (2) use of the body roll, (3) head up at entry, (4) breathing on alternate sides, and (5) high elbow recovery, leading with the hand.[11]

Warm-Up and Workout Structure

Dry land warm-up drills are recommended before practice sessions and should involve shoulder and neck flexibility exercises. Practice should consist of an easy swimming period at the beginning of practice, rest periods during workout to do flexibility exercises, and an easy swim period at the end of practice.[11]

Flexibility

Flexibility can be improved by proprioceptive neuromuscular facilitation. One technique that can be used is described by Holt (1973). This technique (1) stretches passively the affected muscles by slow stretch, and (2) initiates isometric contraction before the muscle is stretched, followed by the concentric contraction of the antagonist muscle groups. "Contraction of the antagonists produces reciprocal relaxation of the agonists allowing for more effective stretching."[11] Stretches include (1) horizontal abduction stretch; (2) shoulder depressor stretch; (3) external rotation stretch; (4) flexor and extensor stretch with towel; (5) horizontal abduction; (6) shoulder depressor switch; and (7) internal rotator stretch. Refer to the section on cuff strains and tendinitis for the descriptions and illustrations of the stretching exercises that should be followed for the rehabilitation of this injury.[11]

Strength Training

Strength training should consist of *program 4*, with progression to *program 5*.

Surgery

Dominguez[2] recommends that surgery be considered when conservative treatment for swimmer's shoulder or impingement syndrome has been tried for 12 months but has not proved effective. Coracoacromial ligament resection, alone or combined with acromioplasty, can be effective for some, but not for those associated with glenohumeral subluxations.

Problem: Loss of Motion and Strength

REHABILITATION

Surgery and subsequent immobilization will result in limited range of motion and weakness. The stretching and strengthening exercises described in the section on rotator cuff injuries (programs 3 and 4) can be performed.

Strength Exercises

Exercises should strengthen the subscapularis and infraspinatus muscles. Internal and external rotation exercises can be performed with rubber tubing, weights, or isometrics.[9]

Rehabilitation *program 4* described previously should be followed by the isotonic program (*program 2*) described and illustrated in the section on rotator cuff tendinitis, and by exercises with Nautilus (see *program 5*).

Nautilus

The Nautilus strength training system is a superb method of fully reconditioning the shoulder, arm, and trunk muscles. It can be introduced when the injured athlete can perform the isotonic dumbbell exercises comfortably with 7.5 to 10.0 lb and has pain-free motion.

The athlete should be instructed to use the equipment with light resistance so that 12 to 15 repetitions of each exercise are possible (see list). Following the normal set (12 to 15 repetitions) with both arms, another set (12 to 15 repetitions) is performed with the injured arm only. Care must be taken to lighten the resistance to a safe, comfortable load, and good stabilization must be maintained. At times it is necessary to adjust the Nautilus machinery to the individual's particular range of motion. Exercises should be performed only within the pain-free range. This cannot be overemphasized. It is important that this be recognized and that the individual be properly instructed on how to do this. Otherwise, reinjury is possible.

Program 5: Nautilus

Super Pullover Machine (latissimus dorsi and other torso).—Follow the steps given below.

1. Adjust the seat so that the top of the shoulders are aligned with the axes of the cams.
2. Check to make sure that the appropriate weight is set.
3. Sit in the seat, adjust the seat belt, and depress the foot pedal with both feet. This will raise the elbow pads in front of the body.
4. Place the elbows on the pad and the palms of the hands on the curved portion of the bar.

5. Provide resistance with the elbows and release the foot pedal. Allow the weight to gently pull the arms backward (Fig 8–12,A).
6. Drive with the elbows and lower the bar to the count of two, until it touches the hips/thighs (Fig 8–12,B).
7. Hold the position for the count of two.
8. To the count of four, slowly allow the bar to return to the starting position.
9. Repeat the exercises again, 8 to 12 times.

Double Chest Machine.—*Arm cross machine* (*pectoralis major, deltoids*).—Follow the steps given below.

1. Adjust the seat so that at step 5 the shoulders are aligned with the cams of the machine overhead.
2. Check to make sure that the appropriate weight is set.

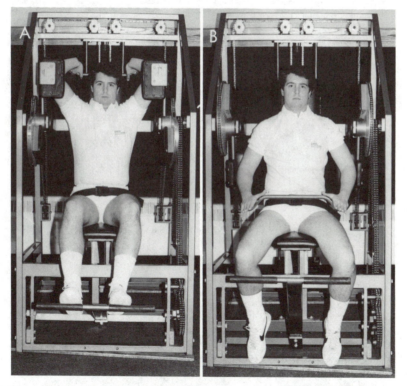

FIG 8–12.
Super pullover machine (latissimus dorsi and other torso). **A,** the starting position for the pullover exercise. Adjust the height of the seat so that the top of the shoulders are aligned with the axes of the cams. Set the appropriate weight. While sitting in the machine with the back straight and the seat belt fastened, raise the elbow pads in front of the body by pushing with both feet on the foot pedal. Place the elbows on the pad, and the hands on the curved portion of the bar. Provide resistance with the elbows and release the foot pedal. Allow the weight to gently pull the arms backward. **B,** the bar is lowered to the hip-thigh area, where it is held for two counts. This position can be reached by driving forward with the elbows from position **A.** After holding this position for two counts, return slowly to the count of four to the starting position. Keep the palms open while performing this exercise. Repeat 8 to 12 times.

3. Fasten the seat belt.
4. With a straight back, and the head back, put the forearms behind the pads, and place the palms of the hands against the handle (Fig 8–13,A).
5. Apply pressure against the pads with the forearms and push forward to the count of two, until the arms come together in front. Hold this position for two counts (Fig 8–13,B).
6. To the count of four, slowly return the arms to the starting position.
7. Repeat 8 to 12 repetitions. Then proceed to the next exercise.

Decline press (chest, shoulder, triceps).—Follow the steps given below.

1. Leave the seat adjusted as for the arm cross exercise.
2. Raise the handles into the starting position by depressing the foot pad with both feet.
3. Place the palms of the hands behind the handles. Keep the back straight, and flat against the back, and keep the head back (Fig 8–14,A).

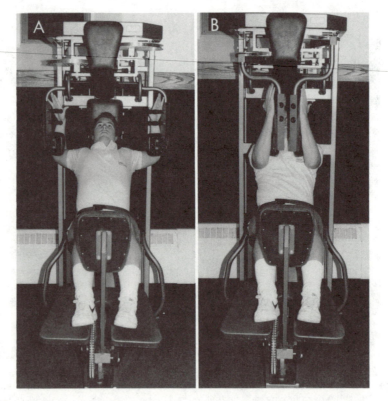

FIG 8–13.
Double chest machine—arm cross (pectoralis major, deltoids). **A,** the starting position for the arm cross exercise. Adjust the seat so that when in position **B,** the shoulders are directly beneath the overhead cams, and fasten the seat belt. With the back straight and the head against the seat back, place the elbows behind the arm pads, and place the palms of the hands on the handles. **B,** apply pressure against the pads with the forearms and push forward to the count of two, until reaching the position shown. Hold this position for two counts, and then slowly return, to the count of four, to the starting position. Repeat 8 to 12 times.

4. Press the bars forward, to the count of two, until the arms are almost but not completely extended. Keep the elbows up while doing this (Fig 8–14,B). Hold this position for two counts.
5. To the count of four, return slowly to the starting position. Repeat 8 to 12 times.

Behind-the-Neck Machine.—Follow the steps given below.

1. Adjust the seat so that the shoulders are aligned with the cams of the machine.
2. Sit straight, with the back flat against the back, and fasten the seat belt.
3. Cross the forearms over the head and place the backs of the upper arms between the rollers (Fig 8–15,A).
4. Apply pressure with the arms against the rollers, lowering them to the count of two, until they touch the torso. Keep the elbows flexed to 90 degrees and the forearms parallel to the wall behind. Hold this position for two counts (Fig 8–15,B).

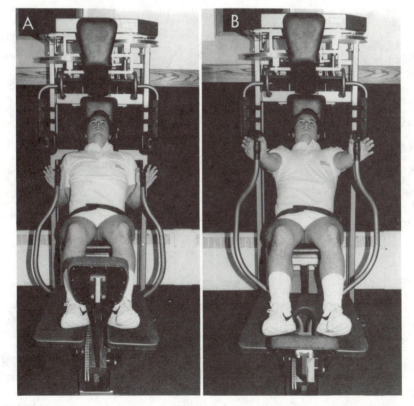

FIG 8–14.
Decline press (chest, shoulders, triceps). **A,** the starting position for the decline press. The seat should remain adjusted as in Fig 8–13. Raise the handles into the starting position by depressing the foot pad with both feet. Place the palms of the hands behind the handles. Keep the back flat and the head back. **B,** the extended position. This can be reached by pressing the bars forward until the arms are almost but not completely extended. Keep the elbows up. Hold this position for two counts, and then slowly lower—to the count of four—to the starting position. Repeat 8 to 12 times.

5. Slowly return to the starting position, taking four counts to do so.
6. Repeat 8 to 12 times at the appropriate weight.

Rowing (Deltoids and Trapezius).—Follow the steps given below.

1. Enter the machine, and sit with the back straight and flat against the back of the machine. Use additional pads between the torso and the front padding if necessary.
2. Place the arms between the rollers, cross one over top of the other, and flex the elbows to 90 degrees (Fig 8–16,A).
3. Drive with the elbows, and apply pressure against the pads, pushing them backward as far as possible. Keep the elbows flexed to 90 degrees and the forearms parallel to the floor. Hold this position for two counts (Fig 8–16,B).
4. Slowly return, to the starting position, taking four counts to do so.
5. Repeat 8 to 12 times.

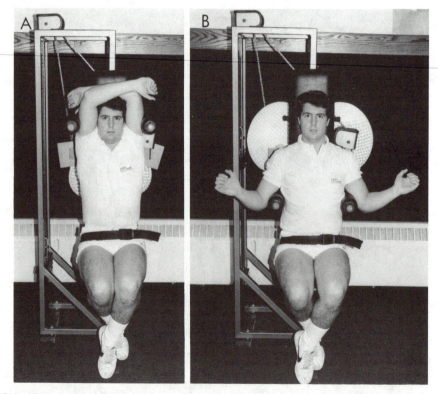

FIG 8–15.
Behind-the-neck machine (latissimus dorsi). **A,** the starting position. Adjust the seat so that the shoulders are aligned with the cams of the machines. Sit up straight and fasten the seat belt. Cross the forearms over the head and place the back of the upper arms between the rollers. **B,** apply pressure with the arms against the rollers, lowering them to the count of two, until they touch the sides of the torso. Keep the elbows flexed to 90 degrees and the forearms parallel to the wall behind. Hold for two counts, then slowly return—to the count of four—to the starting position. Repeat 8 to 12 times at the appropriate weight.

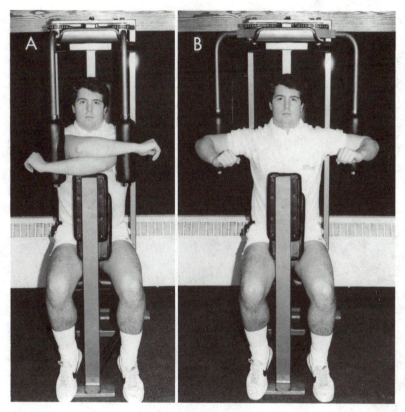

FIG 8–16.
Rowing machine (deltoids, trapezius). **A,** the starting position for rowing. Sit up straight with the back flat against the back of the machine, and use additional pads as necessary. Place the arms between the rollers and cross one over top of the other, and flex the elbows to 90 degrees, as shown. **B,** drive with the elbows, applying pressure against the pads, pushing them back as far as possible. Keep the elbows flexed to 90 degrees and the forearms parallel to the floor. Hold the position shown for two counts, then slowly return to the count of four, to the starting position. Repeat 8 to 12 times.

Double Shoulder Machine.—*Lateral raise* (Deltoids).—Follow the steps given below.

1. Adjust the seat so that the tops of the shoulders are aligned with the cams of the machine.
2. Sit up straight; keep the head back, and fasten the seat belt.
3. Place the hands behind the pads and rest the palms on the handles (Fig 8–17,A).
4. Abduct the arms away from the body, leading with the elbows. Raise the arms to the count of two until the arms are parallel to the floor. Hold this position for two counts (Fig 8–17,B).
5. To the count of four, slowly lower the arms to the starting position.
6. Repeat 8 to 12 times.

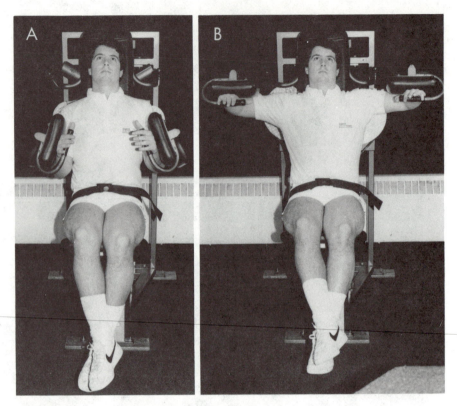

FIG 8–17.
Double shoulder machine, lateral raise (deltoids). **A,** the starting position for the lateral raise. Adjust the seat so that the tops of the shoulders are aligned with the axes of the cams of the machine. Sit up straight, keep the head back, and fasten the seat belt. Place the hands behind the pads and rest the palms on the handles, as shown. **B,** the fully abducted position. From **A,** abduct the arms away from the body, leading with the elbows. Raise the arms to the count of two until the arms are parallel with the floor. Hold this position for two counts, then slowly return to the count of four to the starting position. Repeat 8 to 12 times.

Overhead press (Deltoids, Trapezius).—Follow the steps given below.

1. With the seat adjusted as for the lateral raise, and with the back straight, head back, and seat belt fastened, grasp the handles located just above either shoulder (Fig 8–18,A).
2. Press the handles up over the head until the arms are extended. This should take two counts. Hold this position for two counts. Keep the back pressed flat against the back pad while performing this exercise. *Do not arch* (Fig 8–18,B)!
3. To the count of four, slowly lower the handles to the starting position.
4. Repeat 8 to 12 times.

The shoulder should not be placed in a compromised position if surgery has not been performed.[13] Progress will be slower, atrophy will be greater, and range of motion will be more limited if there has been extensive damage.

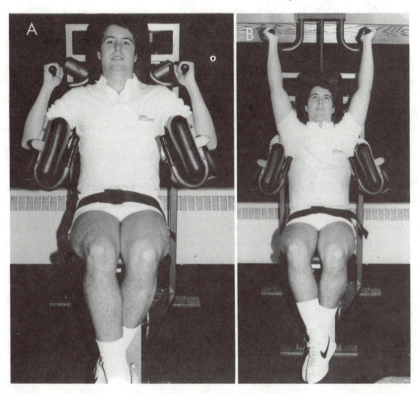

FIG 8–18.
Overhead press (deltoids, triceps). **A,** the starting position for the overhead press. Begin with the seat adjusted as in **A** and **B.** Grasp the handles as shown. Keep the head back. **B,** the fully extended position. Press the handles overhead until the arms are extended (two counts). Hold for 2 seconds, then lower slowly to the count of four. Keep the back pressed flat against the back pad while performing this exercise. *Do not arch!*

REFERENCES

1. Claessens H, Snoeck H: Tendinitis of the long head of the biceps brachii. *Acta Orthop Belg* 1972; 58:124–128.
2. Dominguez RH: Shoulder pain in swimmers. *Phys Sports Med* 1980; 8(7):37–42.
3. Gordon EJ: Diagnoses and treatment of common shoulder disorders. *Med Trial Tech Q* 1981 (Summer); 28:25–37.
4. Greninger LO: Rehabilitation of the glenohumeral joint. *Am Corrective Therapy J* 1977; 31:35–40.
5. Hawkins RJ, Kennedy JC: Impingement syndromes in athletes. *Am J Sports Med* 1980; 8(3):151–158.
6. Henry JH, Genung JA: Natural history of glenohumeral dislocation—revisited. *Am J Sports Med* 1982; 10(3):135–137.
7. Jobe FW, Jobe CM: Painful athletic injuries of the shoulder. *Clin Orthop* 1983; 173:117–124.
8. Kulund DN: The shoulder, in Kulund DN (ed): *The Injured Athlete.* Philadelphia, JB Lippincott Co, 1982, pp 259–294.
9. Matsen FA, Kirby RM: Office evaluation and management of shoulder pain. *Orthop Clin North Am* 1982; 13:453–475.

10. MacNab I: The painful shoulder due to rotator cuff tendinitis. *RI Med J* 1971; 54:367–388.

11. Norgrove-Penny J, Smith C: The prevention and treatment of swimmer's shoulder. *Can J Appl Sport Sci* 1980; 5:195–202.

12. Norwood LA, Terry GC: Shoulder posterior subluxation. *Am J Sports Med* 1984; 12(1):25–30.

13. O'Donoghue DH: Injuries of the shoulder girdle, in O'Donaghue DH (ed): *Treatment of Injuries to Athletes*. Philadelphia, WB Saunders, 1984, pp 118–214.

14. Post M, Silver R, Singh M: Rotator cuff tear: Diagnosis and treatment. *Clin Orthop* 1983; 173:78–91.

15. Penny JN, Smith C: The prevention and treatment of swimmer's shoulder. *Can J Appl Sports Sci* 1980; 5:195–202.

16. Penny JN, Welsh RP: Shoulder impingement syndromes in athletes and their surgical management. *Am J Sports Med* 1981; 9(1):11–15.

17. Rocks JA: Intrinsic shoulder pain syndrome: Rationale for heating and cooling in treatment. *Phys Ther* 1979; 59:153–159.

18. Rothman RH, Parks WW: The vascular anatomy of the rotator cuff. *Clin Orthop* 1965; 41:176–186.

19. Wolfgang GL: Rupture of the musculotendinous cuff of the shoulder. *Clin Orthop* 1978; 134:230–243.

CHAPTER 9

The Neck

Football, diving, wrestling, ice hockey, surfing, equestrian events and gymnastics are activities in which injuries to the cervical spine most frequently occur. Proper treatment and rehabilitation recommendations depend on an accurate identification of the anatomic structures involved, and correct assessment of the severity of the injury.

Injuries to the cervical spine can be discussed according to a classification system that divides them into five groups: mild, moderate, severe, very severe, and catastrophic.[9]

CLASS 1: MILD INJURIES

This category includes stable sprains, strains, and nerve root/brachial plexus neurapraxia. Recovery from mild sprains and strains usually occurs without a specific treatment protocol.

CLASS 2: MODERATE INJURIES

Class 2 includes "occult" fractures, vertebral body compression fractures, disk-space narrowing, degenerative changes due to repeated microtrauma, and grade 2 brachial plexus axonotmesis injuries. In a study of 75 college freshman football recruits at the University of Iowa, by Albright et al.,[1] 32% had one or more of the above lesions as a result of high school injuries.

CLASS 3: SEVERE INJURIES

Severe injuries include unstable lesions with subluxation, dislocation, or fractures without neurological involvement.[9]

CLASS 4: VERY SEVERE INJURIES

Cervical spine injuries with neurological deficits (i.e., fracture/dislocation of the cervical spine) are classified as very severe. In instances in which a partial cord lesion exists, care must be taken so that the lesion does not become complete.[9]

CLASS 5: CATASTROPHIC

Injury to the cervical spine with associated permanent quadriplegia or death can be considered nothing less than a catastrophe.[9]

EMERGENCY MANAGEMENT

Treatment recommendations begin with instructions on how to move the player from the playing field to the hospital. Football helmets should not be removed and pillows should not be placed under the head. This is to ensure that the head and neck remained aligned with the axial skeleton. This alignment is a major consideration when attempts to move the player are made. The basic principle in moving an unconscious player, or one suspected of having a cervical spine injury, is that he be "rolled like a log" onto a spine board. Once the individual is on the board, immobilization of the spine must be maintained.[9]

CLASS 1 INJURY: ACUTE CERVICAL SPRAIN SYNDROME

An acute cervical sprain is an injury frequently seen in contact sports; the patient complains of having "jammed" his neck, with subsequent pain localized to the cervical area. Characteristically, the patient presents with limitation of cervical spine motion without radiation of pain or paresthesia.[10] Neurologic examination is negative and roentgenograms are normal.[10]

In the absence of findings other than pain and limitation of neck motion, identifying the exact nature of the injury may be difficult or impossible. However, it is assumed that either the intervertebral disk structures, ligamentous supporting structures, or the joints between the articular processes have been injured.[10]

In general, treatment of athletes with "cervical sprains" should be tailored to the degree of severity. Immobilizing the neck in a soft collar and using analgesics and anti-inflammatory agents until there is a full, spasm-free range of neck motion is appropriate. If the patient has severe pain and muscle spasm of the cervical spine, hospitalization and the head-halter traction may be indicated. It should be emphasized that individuals with a history of collision injury, pain, and lack of normal range of cervical motion should have routine cervical spine roentgenographic study. Also, lateral flexion and extension roentgenograms are indicated after the acute symptoms subside.[10]

CLASS 1 INJURY: GRADE 1 BRACHIAL PLEXUS NEURAPRAXIA

Included among class 1 injuries are grade 1 brachial plexus, or pinch/stretch neurapraxias of the nerve roots.[4] These injuries are characterized by a sharp, burning pain. It can be felt in the neck, and radiates to the shoulder, arm, and hand. Associated weakness and paresthesia are additional symptoms. The key to the nature of the lesion is its short duration and persistence of full, pain-free range of neck motion.[9] An additional characteristic includes tenderness in the trapezius muscle, usually in the upper middle portion.[4] Motor and sensory function usually return to normal in a few days.[4] Injuries of greater severity can be suspected when paresthesia and/or weakness associated with a limitation of cervical spine motion is present.

Problem: Weakness and Decreased Motion

While range of motion may not be limited, loss of strength will be a problem. Refer to the rehabilitation program at the end of the chapter for descriptions and illustrations of manual resistance exercises and isotonic Nautilus exercises.

CLASS 2 INJURY: GRADE 2 BRACHIAL PLEXUS AXONOTMESIS

These injuries are caused by a stretching of the plexus as the head and cervical spine are forced laterally away from the symptomatic arm and shoulder, usually as a result of a shoulder tackle or fall. Acromioclavicular or glenohumeral pain is usually not present. Paralysis, numbness, and burning sensations in the hands are experienced.[2]

Problem: Weakness

Loss of strength is a major problem resulting from this injury. Grade 2 injuries are characterized by weakness of shoulder abduction, elbow flexion, and external humeral rotation, due to weakening of the deltoid, biceps and infraspinatus.[9, 2] There may also be weakness of triceps, wrist extensors, and grip strength.[2] Strength loss in grade 2 injuries tends to last somewhat longer than in grade 1 brachial plexus injuries; 80% to 90% strength may not be seen for six weeks, and full strength may take as long as six months to be regained.[4]

Treatment can include a light-weight rehabilitation program, with gradual progression to a full shoulder rehabilitation program, and eventual return to activity. Neck rehabilitation exercises are described at the end of the chapter. For strengthening exercises for the shoulder, biceps, triceps, and wrist, refer to the rehabilitation program described in Chapters 8, 10, and 11.

The athlete may return to competition if there is no observable pain or weakness when he/she is tested against resistance through the full range of motion.[4] Individuals with this injury should not be permitted to compete until full strength returns.[9] This is assessable through comparison of weight-lifting ability to the preseason baseline measurements, and comparison of the strength of the injured extremity to that of the uninjured extremity. This can be done, for example, on the abduction machine.[2] It is important to be alert to possible fractures, although this is not likely.[4]

Preventive measures should be implemented so that these injuries can be avoided. Included are (1) allowing individuals to participate only in activities appropriate for their height and weight, (2) requiring neck strengthening exercises, (3) using the proper equipment, padding, and playing techniques and (4) using cervical collars.[2] Manual resistance and Nautilus exercises should be performed on a year-round basis.

PERIPHERAL NERVE INJURIES

Peripheral nerve injuries[10] may involve the spinal accessory nerve (trapezius muscle), the suprascapular nerve (the supraspinatus, the infraspinatus, and the teres major muscles), the axillary nerve (deltoid and teres minor muscles), and the long thoracic nerve (serratus anterior muscles).

The spinal accessory nerve is vulnerable anteriorly, just proximal to its entrance into the undersurface of the trapezius, approximately 1 in. above the clavicle. It can be injured by a direct blow from a hockey or a lacrosse stick, or a shoulder pad could be forced against it. With significant trauma, there may be weakness when lifting the arm or shrugging the shoulders, and there may be a rotary winging of the scapula. This injury should be followed up by electromyography. If there is no recovery within six months, the nerve should be explored surgically.

The suprascapular nerve may be injured by a direct blow to the base of the neck. This causes shoulder weakness, which is noticeable at 90 degrees of abduction. This injury must be differentiated from a resolving grade 2 brachial plexus injury. In follow-up of grade 2 brachial plexus injuries we have noted that the biceps and deltoid functions return to normal significantly faster than the supraspinatus and infraspinatus. Hence, a grade II plexus injury, if seen late, may readily appear as an isolated suprascapular nerve injury. Careful questioning and electromyographic evaluation often help differentiate between the two. This differential diagnosis is particularly important since suprascapular nerve injury without significant return of strength after six months may warrant surgical exploration.

Without a concomitant shoulder dislocation, an axillary nerve injury is an uncommon finding.

Wing scapula, or serratus anterior paralysis, results from traction injury to the long thoracic nerve of Bell. Initially the injury is characterized by mild pain radiating through the neck to the scapula, and is caused by either a single incident of trauma or repeated activity. Eventually, after a few weeks, range of motion, specifically abduction and forward flexion, becomes limited, weakness develops, and activity becomes limited. The injury has visible characteristics as well. While standing, the medial and inferior borders of the scapula appear closer to the spine than those of the scapula on the unaffected side. Winging can be observed when the patient flexes the shoulder forward to 90 degrees, externally rotates the joint while extending the elbow, and presses against a wall.[5]

The mechanism for the injury, as proposed by Gregg et al.,[5] is as follows: the head is rotated, flexed and tilted laterally away from the involved shoulder; the nerve is pulled anteriorly and medially. When the ipsilateral arm is raised overhead, the distal fixation point in the muscle mass of the superior serratus anterior moves posteriorly, laterally, and inferiorly, thereby exerting a pathological stretch on the long thoracic nerve. This mechanism is based on anatomical studies in laboratory as well as on clinical observations.

Gregg et al.[5] also propose a course of treatment for wing scapula. This includes rest, followed by graduated range of motion exercises. Pendulum exercises, passive stretching of the latissimus dorsi and pectoralis muscles, as well as range of motion for the trapezius, rhomboids, and levator scapula are to be included. A graduated course of strengthening exercises, progressing from wall push-ups to floor push-ups, chin-ups and military presses can begin when range of motion has been regained. Surgery is only advocated if a return to function has not occurred after two years.

Several months after the injury occurs it may be difficult to distinguish between a partially recovered brachial plexus injury and a peripheral nerve injury. An awareness of the clinical manifestations and the electromyographic findings at serial intervals may help to differentiate between the two entities.[10]

CLASS 3 AND 4 INJURIES: FRACTURES AND/OR DISLOCATIONS

Fractures and/or dislocations of the cervical spine may be stable or unstable, and may or may not be associated with neurological deficit. When fracture or disruption of the soft-tissue supporting structure immediately violates or threatens to violate the integrity of the spinal cord, implementation of certain management and treatment principles is imperative.[10]

The first goal is to protect the spinal cord and nerve roots from injury through mismanagement. It has been estimated that 50% of neurologic deficits occur after the initial injury. That is, if a patient with an unstable lesion is carelessly manipulated when being transported to a medical facility or subsequently inappropriately managed, further encroachment on the spinal cord can occur.[10]

Second, traumatic malalignment of the cervical spine should be reduced as quickly and gently as possible. This will effectively decompress the spinal cord. When dislocation or anterior angulation and translation are demonstrated roentgenographically, immediate reduction is attempted with skull traction utilizing Gardner-Wells tongs. These tongs can be easily and rapidly applied under local anesthesia, without shaving the head, in the emergency room or in the patient's bed. They are spring-loaded, thus precluding the necessity for drilling the outer table of the skull. The tongs are attached to a cervical-traction pulley and weight is added in 5-lb increments every 15 minutes, using the rule of thumb of 5 lb per disk level up to 25 to 40 lb for lower cervical injury. Reduction is substantiated by a lateral roentgenogram obtained 15 minutes after each addition of weight.[10]

Unilateral facet dislocations, particularly at the C3–4 level, are not always reducible using skeletal traction. Such traumatic malalignment of the cervical spine should be reduced as quickly as possible, but if skeletal traction is not possible, manipulative or open reduction under general anesthesia should be effected.

It has been proposed that the presence of a bulbocavernous reflex indicates that spinal shock has worn off, and that except for recovery of an occasional nerve root at the level of injury, the paralysis, both motor and sensory, does not recover regardless of treatment. The bulbocavernous reflex is produced by a pulling on the urethral catheter, which stimulates the trigone of the bladder, producing a reflex contraction of the anal sphincter around the examiner's gloved finger. Although the presence of a bulbocavernous reflex is generally a sign that there will be no further neurologic recovery below the level of injury, this is not always completely accurate. The presence of this reflex should not give the clinician license to handle the situation in an elective fashion. Cervical spine subluxations and dislocations associated with quadriparesis should be reduced as quickly as possible, by whatever means necessary, if maximal recovery is to be expected.[10]

Regarding the role of operative decompression for cervical fractures and/or dislocations, we believe there is a limited role for cervical laminectomy in their treatment. Only rarely, when excision of foreign bodies or bony fragments in the spinal canal is necessary, is a posterior laminectomy indicated. Realignment of the spine is the most effective method for decompression of the cervical cord.

In most instances in which a vertebral body burst fracture is associated with anterior compression of the cord, decompression is logically effected through an anterior approach with corpectomy and interbody fusion. Likewise, traumatic intervertebral disk herniation with cord involvement is best managed through an anterior diskectomy and interbody fusion.[10]

Indications for surgical decompression of the spinal cord have been delineated. A documented increase in neurologic signs is the clearest mandate for surgical decompression. Further observation, expectancy, and procrastination in this situation are contraindicated. Persistent partial cord or root signs, with objective evidence of clinical compression, is also an indication for surgical intervention.[10]

Preceding and following reduction of cervical spine fractures and/or dislocations, the use of parenteral corticosteroids (dexamethasone) to decrease the inflammatory reactions of the injured cord and surrounding soft-tissue structures is very important. Drugs that inhibit norepinephrine synthesis or deplete catecholamines have been advocated to prevent autodigestion of the cord. However, there is no evidence as yet that this is of value in altering prognosis of cord recovery. Procedures such as durotomy, myelotomy, and rhizotomy require extensive laminectomy, adding further instability to the spine, and are contraindicated.[10]

The third goal in managing fractures and/or dislocations of the cervical spine is to effect rapid and secure stability to prevent residual deformity and instability with associated pain, and the possibility of further trauma to the neural elements. The method of immobilization depends on the postreduction status of the injury. Thompson et al.[8] have concisely delineated indications for nonsurgical and surgical methods for achieving stability. These concepts[10] for managing cervical spine fractures and dislocations may be summarized as follows:

1. Patients with stable compression fractures of the vertebral body, undisplaced fractures of the lamina or lateral masses, or soft-tissue injuries without detectable neurologic deficit can be adequately treated with traction and subsequent protection by using a cervical brace until healing occurs.

2. Stable, reduced facet dislocations without neurological deficit can also be treated conservatively in a Halo jacket until healing had been demonstrated by negative lateral flexion-extension roentgenograms.

3. Unstable cervical spine fractures or fracture dislocations without neurological deficit may require surgical methods to ensure stability.

4. Absolute indications for surgical stabilization of an unstable injury without neurological deficit are late instability following closed treatment, and flexion-rotation injuries with unreduced locked facet.

5. Relative indications for surgical stabilizations in unstable injuries without neurological deficit are anterior subluxation greater than 20%, certain atlantoaxial fractures or dislocations, and unreduced vertical compression injuries with neck flexion.

6. Cervical spine fractures with complete cord lesion require reduction followed by stabilization by closed or open means as indicated.

7. Cervical spine fractures with incomplete cord lesions require reduction followed by careful evaluation for surgical intervention.[8]

The fourth and final goal of treatment is rapid and effective rehabilitation started early in the treatment process.[10]

REHABILITATION PROGRAM

Whether it is used initially as part of a conservative course, or postoperatively, the aim of the rehabilitation program is usually the same, namely to restore range of motion, and adequate strength.

The rehabilitation program can begin with range of motion exercises followed by isometric resistance, and finally progress to isotonic exercises as the physician sees fit. Isometric contractions should be held for 6 seconds, then relaxed. Three sets of six repetitions should be performed. These exercises are performed against resistance, provided either by the individuals own hands, a towel, or a partner's hands.[6] See Chapter 5 for further discussion of Nautilus.

Range of Motion

Neck Flexion.—While standing or sitting, flex the neck forward and attempt to touch the chin to the chest. Hold this position for 10 to 15 seconds; relax and repeat six to ten times (Fig 9–1,A).

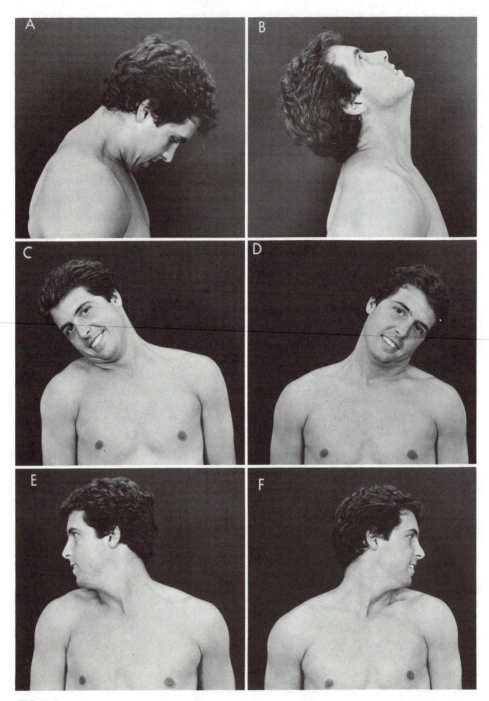

FIG 9–1.
A, neck flexion stretch. While standing or sitting, flex the neck forward and attempt to touch the chin to the chest. Hold this position for 10 to 15 seconds; relax and repeat. **B,** neck extension stretch. While standing or sitting, extend the neck backward and attempt to touch the back of the head to the upper back. Hold for 10 to 15 seconds; relax and repeat. **C,** lateral bend stretch to the right. *(Continued.)*

Neck Extension.—While standing or sitting, extend the neck backward and attempt to touch the back of the head to the upper back. Hold for 10 to 15 seconds; relax and repeat six to ten times (Fig 9–1,B).

Lateral Bending (Right).—While standing or sitting, look straight ahead. Bend the neck to the right, and attempt to touch the right ear to the top of the right shoulder. There should be a stretch on the left side of the neck. Hold the stretch for 10 to 15 seconds; relax, and repeat six to ten times (Fig 9–1,C).

Lateral Bending (Left).—While standing or sitting, look straight ahead. Bend the neck to the left and attempt to touch the left ear to the top of the left shoulder. There should be a stretch on the right side of the neck. Hold the stretch for 10 to 15 seconds; relax and repeat. Repeat six to ten times (Fig 9–1,D).

Lateral Rotation (Right).—While standing or sitting, look straight ahead. Rotate the head to the right and try to touch the chin to the right shoulder. Hold the stretch for 10 to 15 seconds; relax and repeat six to ten times (Fig 9–1,E).

Lateral Rotation (Left).—While standing or sitting, look straight ahead. Rotate the head to the left and try to touch the chin to the left shoulder. Hold the stretch for 10 to 15 seconds; relax and repeat six to ten times. (Fig 9–1,F).

Isometric Resistance

Strength can be improved initially with isometric resistance exercises. These exercises help to strengthen the muscles of the neck without moving the neck through the range of motion.

Neck Flexion.—Place the palms of both hands on the forehead. While providing resistance with the hands, try to press the forehead forward, without actually moving it. Hold for 6 seconds. Relax and repeat six to ten times (Fig 9–2,A).

Neck Extension.—With the head flexed slightly forward, place the palms of the hands against the back of the head. While providing resistance with the hands, try to push the head backward, without actually moving it. Hold for 6 seconds. Relax and repeat six to ten times (Fig 9–2,B).

FIG 9–1 (cont.).
While standing or sitting, look straight ahead. Bend the neck to the right, and attempt to touch the right ear to the top of the right shoulder. There should be a stretch on the left side of the neck. Hold the stretch for 10 to 15 seconds; relax and repeat. **D,** lateral bend to the left. Begin sitting or standing and look straight ahead. Bend the neck to the left and attempt to touch the left ear to the top of the left shoulder. There should be a stretch on the right side of the neck. Hold the stretch for 10 to 15 seconds; relax and repeat. **E,** lateral rotation to the right. Begin standing or sitting. Rotate the head to the right and try to touch the chin to the right shoulder. Hold the stretch for 10 to 15 seconds; relax and repeat. **F,** lateral rotation to the left. Begin standing or sitting. Rotate the head to the left and try to touch the chin to the left shoulder. Hold the stretch for 10 to 15 seconds; relax and repeat.

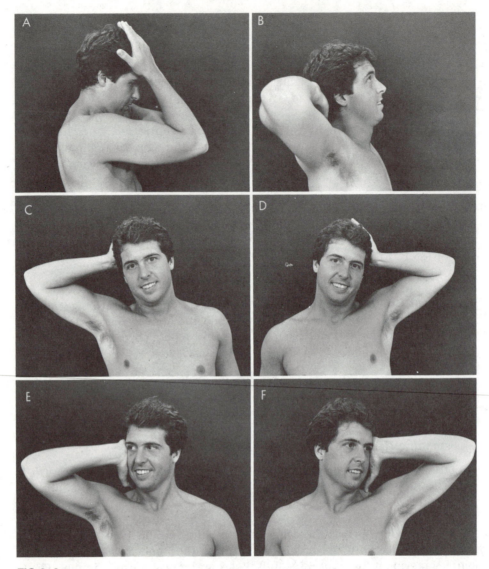

FIG 9–2.

Isometric resistance exercises. **A,** neck flexion against isometric resistance. While standing or sitting, place the palms of both hands on the forehead. While providing resistance with both hands, press forward. The head should not move. Contract for 6 seconds; relax and repeat. **B,** neck extension against isometric resistance. While standing or sitting, place the palms of both hands against the back of the head. While providing resistance with the hands, try to push the head backward. The head should not move. Contract for 6 seconds; relax and repeat. **C,** lateral bending to the right against isometric resistance. Place the right hand against the side of the head. While providing resistance with one hand, try to move the head (right ear) toward the right shoulder. The head should not move. Contract for 6 seconds; relax and repeat. **D,** lateral bending to the left against isometric resistance. Place the left hand against the side of the head. While providing resistance with the one hand, try to move the head (left ear) toward the left shoulder. The head should not move. Contract for 6 seconds; relax and repeat. **E,** lateral rotation to the right against isometric resistance. Place the right hand against the temple. Apply pressure with the right hand and try to rotate the head to the right. Try to touch the chin to the right shoulder. The head should not move. Contract for 6 seconds; relax and repeat. **F,** lateral rotation to the right against isometric resistance. Place the left hand against the temple. Apply pressure with the left hand and try to rotate the head to the left. Try to touch the chin to the left shoulder. The head should not move. Contract for 6 seconds; relax and repeat.

Lateral Bending.—Place the right hand against the side of the head. While providing resistance with the hand, try to move the head to the right shoulder. The head should not move. Hold the position for 6 seconds; relax and repeat six to ten times (Fig 9–2,C). Repeat the exercise for the opposite side (Fig 9–2,D).

Lateral Rotation (Right).—Place the right hand against the temple. While applying pressure with the right hand, rotate the head to the right, and try to touch the chin to the right shoulder. The head should not move. Hold the position for 6 seconds; relax and repeat six to ten times (Fig 9–2,E).

Lateral Rotation (Left).—Place the left hand against the temple. While applying pressure with the left hand, rotate the head to the left and try to touch the chin to the left shoulder. The head should not move. Hold the position for 6 seconds; relax and repeat six to ten times (Fig 9–2,F).

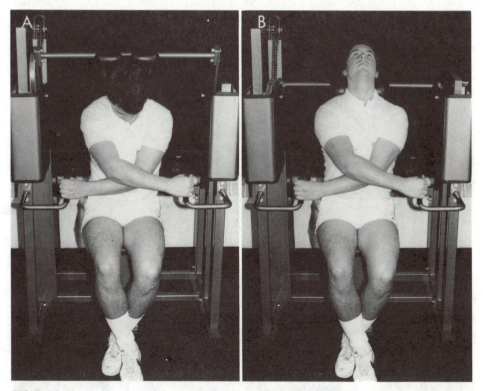

FIG 9–3.
Nautilus four-way neck extension. **A,** starting position for posterior extension on the Nautilus four-way neck machine. With the seat properly adjusted, sit in the machine so that the back of the head is touching the pads. The neck will be flexed forward so that the chin is touching the chest. Cross both arms in front and grasp both handles to either side. **B,** full posterior extension. From the position in **A,** press the head backward against the pads and extend it back as far as possible. Hold this position for 2 seconds. Slowly return to the count of four to the starting position. Relax and repeat 8 to 12 times.

Manual Resistance

Manual resistance is an effective method of strengthening the neck musculature when the athlete is able to work through a comfortable range of motion. Resistance is applied in the same manner as that used for isometric strengthening; however, the head is allowed to move through the range of available range of motion while resistance is applied manually.

Isotonic Exercise

An isotonic exercise program can often follow the isometric or manual resistance program. Wall pulleys can be used for these, as can Universal and Nautilus equipment.[6] Among the exercises that can be performed are flexion, extension, oblique flexion, and extension, as well as shoulder shrugs and high pulls.[6]

Nautilus strength training may be necessary for athletes participating in certain sports, such as football and wrestling, but this level of training is not required for all persons. This kind of rehabilitation program should be performed following the recommendation of a physician.

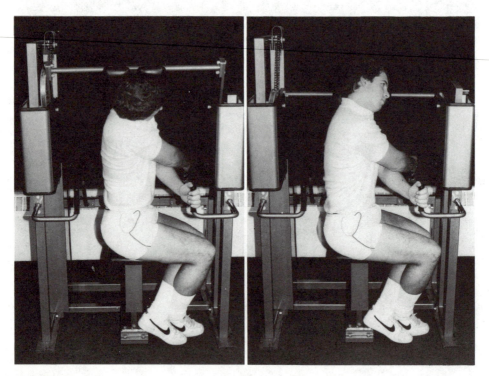

FIG 9–4.
Nautilus four-way neck lateral contraction (side of neck). **A,** starting position for lateral contraction to the left in the Nautilus four-way machine. Sit in the machine with the left ear to the center of the pads. The neck will be laterally contracted fully to the right. Cross both arms in front and grasp the handles on either side. **B,** full lateral contraction to the left. From the position in **A,** move the head from right to left against the pads, until the left ear is as close as possible to the left shoulder. Hold this position for 2 seconds. Keep the shoulders square. Slowly return to the count of four to the starting position. Relax and repeat 8 to 12 times. Repeat this exercise for the opposite (right) side.

Nautilus Four-Way Neck Extension and Flexion

1. With the seat properly adjusted, sit in the machine so that the back of the head is touching the pads. The neck will be flexed forward so that the chin is touching the chest. Cross both arms in front and grasp both handles to either side (Fig 9–3,A).
2. From Step 1, press the head backwards against the pads and extend it back as far as possible. Hold this position for two seconds (Fig 9–3,B). Slowly return to the count of four to the starting position. Relax, and repeat 8-12 times.
3. For neck flexion, sit facing the pads with the forehead against them, and the neck extended. Press forward until the neck is fully flexed. Hold for two seconds. Return to the extended position. Relax and repeat 8–12 times.

Nautilus Four-Way Neck Lateral Contraction (Side of Neck)

1. Sit in the machine with the left ear to the center of the pads. The neck will be laterally contracted fully to the right. Cross both arms in front and grasp the handles on either side (Fig 9–4,A).
2. From final position in step 1, move the head from right to left against the pads, until the left ear is as close as possible to the left shoulder. Hold this position for 2 seconds. Keep the shoulders square (Fig 9–4,B). Slowly return to the count of four to the starting position. Relax and repeat 8 to 12 times.

REFERENCES

1. Albright JP, et al: Nonfatal cervical spine injuries in interscholastic football. *JAMA* 1976; 236:1243.
2. Archembault JL: Brachial plexus stretch injury. *J Am Coll Health* 1983; 31:256–260.
3. Bruce DA, Schut L, Sutton LN: Brain and cervical spine injuries occurring during organized sports activities in children and adolescents. *Primary Care* 1984; 11:175–194.
4. Clancy WG: Brachial plexus and upper extremity peripheral nerve injuries, in Torg JS (ed): *Athletic Injuries to the Head, Neck, and Face*. Philadelphia, Lea & Febiger Inc, 1982, pp 215–220.
5. Gregg JR, Labosky D, Harty M, et al: Serratus anterior paralysis in the young. *J Bone Joint Surg* 1979; 61A:825–831.
6. Kulund DN: Athletic injuries to the head, face, and neck, in Kulund DN (ed): *The Injured Athlete*. Philadelphia, JB Lippincott Co, 1982, pp 225–257.
7. O'Donaghue DH: Injuries of the spine, in O'Donaghue DH (ed): *Treatment of Injuries to Athletes*. Philadelphia, WB Saunders Co, 1984, pp 362–387.
8. Thompson RC, et al: Current concepts in management of cervical fractures and dislocations. *Am J Sports Med* 1975; 3:159.
9. Torg JS: Athletic injuries to the cervical spine. *Surgical Rounds*, November 1978, pp 40–50.
10. Torg JS, Wiesel SW, Rothman RH: Diagnosis and management of cervical spine injuries, in Torg JS (ed): *Athletic Injuries to the Head, Neck, and Face*. Philadelphia, Lea & Febiger Inc, 1982, pp 181–209.

CHAPTER 10

The Elbow

INJURY: TRAUMATIC OLECRANON BURSITIS

Traumatic olecranon bursitis is usually caused by a fall on the point of the elbow. It is characterized by hemorrhage into the olecranon bursa.

Treatment consists of early aspiration, use of ice, and compression. Appropriate compression is accomplished by wrapping the entire arm from the hand to axilla with an elastic bandage.

The elbow should be well padded for resumption of activity; otherwise, a chronic problem may develop. In cases of chronic olecranon bursitis, surgical removal of the bursa can be the treatment of choice.[14]

INJURY: IRRITATION OF THE ULNAR NERVE

Irritation of the ulnar nerve occurs infrequently as a result of certain throwing activities, such as pitching a baseball or throwing a javelin. It is characterized by pain and shocking sensation down to the fourth and fifth fingers, and may be associated with transient paresthesia. Late sequelae can include increased numbness along the distribution of the ulnar nerve, and weakness in adduction and abduction of the fingers. Injections are contraindicated. Surgery may be indicated in instances of definite ulnar nerve palsy.[14]

INJURY: STRAINS

Several muscle-tendon units of the elbow are subject to strain. Strain of the triceps tendon at its attachment on the olecranon is characterized by tenderness with pain on forceful extension and full passive flexion. If the injury is acute, there may be local heat, and forceful extension will tend to aggravate the condition. The biceps tendon can also be strained at its attachment below the neck of the radius. The symptoms are often obscured. Complete ruptures of the radial attachment should be treated surgically. The brachialis is susceptible near its attachment to the ulna. Muscle function can be disturbed.

Treatment for acute cases includes ice application, compression, and rest. Immobilization may be warranted in the acute stage.[14] An injury commonly seen in the throwing athlete involves microtears at the origin of the flexor-pronator muscle group. This problem occurs in the fully developed athlete after the medial epicondyle has fused to the humerus. Treatment should consist of rest, steroid injection, and reverse tennis elbow exercises. These include wrist flexor stretching and strengthening exercises (see section on tennis elbow).[15]

INJURY: SPRAIN

Sprains of the elbow are relatively uncommon. They can vary from first- to third-degree injuries. The mechanism of injury differs for various ligaments. The medial collateral ligaments are sprained in much the same manner as those of the knee; a valgus stress is placed on the ligamentous structures. When the force exceeds the elastic capability of the ligament(s), injury results. Repetition of the mechanism of injury results in pain. Instability is infrequent. Symptoms characterizing the injury include: pain and localized tenderness along the medial aspect, and pain on elbow extension.

Treatment for acute ligamentous injuries involves the application of cold, and may include some form of immobilization until painful tenderness and swelling subside.

INJURY: PITCHING INJURIES IN CHILDREN

Although the mechanics of pitching are similar for both child and adult, the injuries produced are quite different.[17] In the child, the bony structures are characterized by the presence of the elements of enchrondral ossification, that is, epiphyses, apophyses, and epiphyseal plates (growth plates). These structures represent the weakest link in the musculoskeletal chain and are easily injured. In the adult, these structures are no longer present and the stresses of pitching are exerted on the ligaments, tendons, and bone.

"Little leaguer's elbow" may be classified as follows:

1. Medial epicondylar apophysitis
   a. Accelerated apophyseal growth with delayed closure of the epicondylar growth plate.
   b. Traction apophysitis with fragmentation of the medial epicondylar apophysis.
   c. Avulsion of the medial epicondylar apophysis.
2. Osteochondrosis of the humeral capitellum.
3. Osteochondrosis of the radial head.

The term "little leaguer's elbow" is used to describe several different problems. Medial epicondylar apophysitis, itself a poor term, can manifest as one of three different clinical and roentgenographic entities.

Accelerated medial apophyseal growth with delayed closure of the medial epicondylar plate is seen in Little Leaguers who have been engaged in repetitive pitching. Generally, the symptoms are minimal and diagnosis is made on the basis of the roentgenogram. This condition does not cause significant disability. If symptoms warrant treatment, simply resting the arm is sufficient.

Traction apophysitis likewise has a classic roentgenographic picture. Again, the cause is repetitive pitching, which can result in pain, swelling, and tenderness over the medial humeral epicondylar apophysis. If symptoms are significant, the arm should be rested.

Complete avulsion of the medial epicondylar apophysis occurs acutely with attempts to throw as hard as possible. Pain, swelling, and tenderness are present over the apophysis. If separation of the apophysis is less than 5 mm, the extremity should be immobilized in plaster for three weeks. If the separation is 5 mm or more, open reduction and internal fixation are indicated.

Osteochondrosis of the radial head is a relatively rare lesion, although Ellman[3] has documented five cases; Adams,[1,2] two; and Tullos and King,[18] one; all occurring in preadolescent pitchers. Characteristically, pain develops in the elbow of the pitching arm and increases with throwing. Clinically, swelling and tenderness are localized over the radial head and there is limitation of extension. On the basis of roentgenographic and histological evidence, Ellman[3] found changes in the radial head similar to those seen in Legg-Calvé-Perthes disease, that is, condensation, fragmentation, and bony restoration with deformity, articular incongruity, and subsequent arthritic changes. Initial treatment consists of immobilization until the acute symptoms subside. Any further pitching is prohibited. If the radial head becomes markedly deformed, excision may be considered after the healing phase has been completed.

Osteochondrosis of the humeral capitulum also occurs in preadolescents who have pitched in Little League. In all probability this is also an aseptic necrosis of the involved area. Again, treatment should be aimed at effecting immobilization during the acute phase, and there should be no pitching until the lesion heals. As with osteochondrosis of the radial head, the process can take a year and a half to run its course. If the fragment dislodges and becomes loose in the elbow joint, surgical removal is indicated.[17]

PITCHING INJURIES: ADULT

There is a series of injuries that can occur from the extensive stress placed on the arm and elbow during pitching. These injuries can be categorized according to anatomical location.

Medial injuries include medial epicondylitis, medial collateral ligament sprain, flexor-pronator strains, compartment injuries, and medial calcific deposits on the medial aspect of the ulna. Medial epicondylitis was discussed previously. Pain in the medial compartments can be caused by valgus extension overload during the acceleration phase of pitching.[5]

Posterior compartment injuries also occur, usually in the follow-through phase of pitching.[5] Among posterior injuries, olecranon impingement is a common problem. It results in heterotrophic bone formation of the olecranon and its fossa. This results in an extension block. Symptoms of olecranon impingement include swelling in the olecranon fossa with associated inflammation. Treatment should consist of surgical removal of the heterotrophic bone.

Ulnar neuritis and ulnar nerve entrapment are two other injuries that can occur. Tingling pain to the fourth and fifth digits of the throwing hand with each pitch indicates ulnar nerve entrapment. Symptoms are more likely to be localized to the elbow area in ulnar neuritis and are more often caused by irritation of the nerve during the pitch.

Pitching injuries can be treated conservatively with the following measures: rest, heat application before activity, ice application after activity, the administration of systemic anti-inflammatory medication (enteric-coated sodium salicylate, indomethacin, oxyphenbutazone, phenylbutazone), physical therapy (whirlpool, ultrasound), attention to technique, and exercises (warm-up and Fungo routine).[5, 19]

Problem: Limited Motion and Weakness

For ulnar nerve irritation, strains, and sprains, the problems requiring attention following immobilization will be limited range of elbow flexion and extension, and flexion and extension weakness. The elbow flexion and extension range of motion exercises (active and active-assisted) described in the rehabilitation program should be performed to improve range of motion. The importance of regaining full elbow extension cannot be overemphasized. Once range of motion has improved, the elbow flexion/biceps curls, and elbow extension/triceps curls should be performed to increase strength. In addition to elbow exercises, wrist exercises are required for the rehabilitation of pitching injuries to both adults and children.

REHABILITATION

Elbow Flexion Exercises

Active.—Flex the elbow as far as possible and hold for 10 seconds. Relax and repeat ten times.

Active-Assisted.—Perform the flexion exercise described above, except as the elbow is flexed, provide assistance by applying pressure with the opposite arm (Fig 10–1,A).

Elbow Extension Exercises

Active.—Extend the elbow as far as possible. Hold for 10 seconds; relax and repeat ten times.

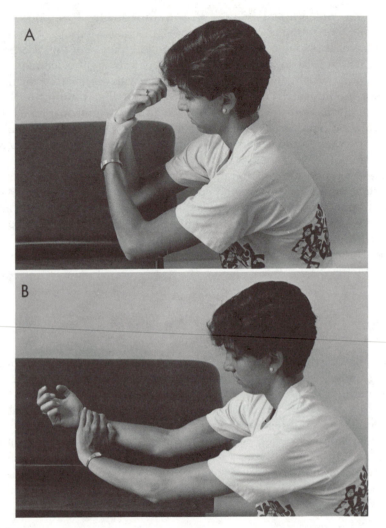

FIG 10–1.
Elbow flexion range of motion/active-assisted. **A,** elbow flexion with assistance. Flex the elbow to 90 degrees and rest it on a flat surface. Provide assistance with the opposite hand and attempt to flex the elbow. **B,** elbow extension with assistance. With the elbow resting on a flat surface, provide assistance with the opposite hand and attempt to extend the elbow.

Active-Assisted.—Perform the extension exercise described above, except as the elbow is extended, provide assistance by applying pressure with the opposite hand (Fig 10–1,B).

Strengthening Exercises

Once range of motion has been regained, it is important to work toward regaining any lost strength. This can be accomplished with isotonic exercises.

Elbow Flexion Exercises (Biceps Curls).—With the upper extremity extended by the side, grasp a dumbbell (weight) in hand. Keeping the elbow and upper arm close to the body, flex the arm, lifting the weight through the range of motion to the fully flexed position (two counts). Hold in this position for two counts, and then lower slowly to the starting position (four counts) (Fig 10–2).

Elbow Extension Exercises (Triceps Curls).—Raise the upper extremity forward until the shoulder is flexed to 180 degrees. Flex the elbow to 90 degrees. Support the elbow with the opposite hand. Grasp a dumbbell (weight) in hand. Holding the elbow close to the head, extend against gravity as much as possible (two counts). Hold the extended position for two counts, and then slowly return to the starting position (four counts). Repeat 8 to 12 times (Fig 10–3).

Strengthening exercises can also be performed on Nautilus machines.

Biceps Curls (Nautilus Biceps Machine).—Adjust the weight. Sit in the seat and align the elbows with the cams of the machine. Use extra padding if necessary. Keep the back straight. With palms up, grasp the bar with both hands at the curved portion (Fig 10–4,A). Raise the weight by pulling the bar to the chin. Hold this position for 2 seconds, then slowly lower to the count of four, to the starting position. Keep the back straight while doing this exercise. Concentrate on pulling with the arms, not the shoulder and back (Fig 10–4,B).

Triceps Extension (Nautilus Triceps Machine).—Set the appropriate weight. Sit in the seat and place the elbows on the pads in front, aligning them with the cams of the machine. Place the hands behind the pads at the shoulders so that the little fingers touch the pads and the thumbs are toward the shoulders. Adjust the padding so that the elbows are slightly higher than the shoulders (Fig 10–5,A). Extend the arms, pushing against the pads with the hands, moving through the range of motion until full extension is reached. Hold this position for 2 seconds, then return slowly to the count of four to the starting position. Concentrate on keeping the elbows on the pads. Repeat 8 to 12 times (Fig 10–5,B).

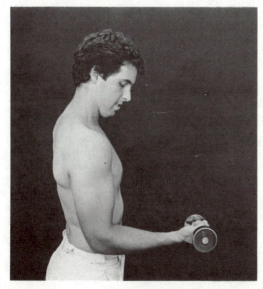

FIG 10–2.
Elbow flexion/biceps curls. The isotonic biceps curl using a dumbbell at 90 degrees flexion. Grasp a dumbbell weight and extend the upper extremity by the side. Keeping the elbow and upper arm close to the body, flex the arm, lifting the weight through the range of motion to the fully flexed position. Hold for 2 seconds, and then lower slowly to the count of 4 seconds to the starting position. Relax. Repeat 8 to 12 times.

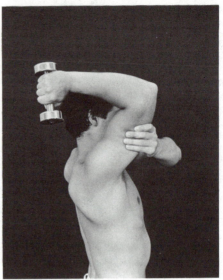

FIG 10–3.
Elbow extension/triceps curl. The isotonic triceps curl using a dumbbell. Raise the arm forward until the shoulder is flexed to 180 degrees. Flex the elbow to 90 degrees and grasp a dumbbell. Support the arm with the opposite hand. While holding the elbow close to the head, extend the elbow against gravity as far as possible, taking 2 seconds to do so. Hold the extended position for 2 seconds and slowly return to the count of four to the starting position.

Wrist Flexor Stretch.—Place the palms of the hands together. Raise the elbows upward, pushing the hands together. Hold this stretched position for 10 seconds. Relax, then repeat six to ten times (see Fig 11–1).

Wrist Extensor Stretch.—Place the backs of the hands together. Lower the elbows to the floor, pushing the hands together. Hold this stretched position for 10 seconds. Relax and repeat six to ten times (see Fig 11–2).

Forearm Flexor Stretching Exercise.—Sit on a stool and rest the arm and elbow, fully extended, on a table. With the opposite hand, actively pull the fingers and wrist into the fully flexed position. Hold for 10 seconds, rest, and repeat. Repeat 10 times (Fig 10–6,A).

Forearm Extensor Stretching Exercise.—Sit on a stool and rest the arm and elbow, fully extended, on a table. With the opposite hand, actively pull the fingers and wrist into the fully extended position. Hold for 10 seconds, rest, and repeat. Repeat 10 times (Fig 10–6,B).

Wrist Flexion Strengthening.—Place the forearm on a flat surface, palm up. Bend the elbow to 90 degrees. Grasp a dumbbell (weight) and allow it to pull the wrist into the fully extended position. Slowly flex the wrist until it is fully flexed. Hold this position for 1 second, then slowly return it to the starting position (Figs 10–7,A and B).

Wrist Extension Strengthening.—Place the forearm on a flat surface, palm down. Bend the elbow to 90 degrees. Grasp a dumbbell (weight) and allow it to pull the wrist into the fully flexed position. Slowly extend the wrist until it is fully extended. Hold this position for 1 second, then slowly return to the starting position (Figs 10–8,A and B).

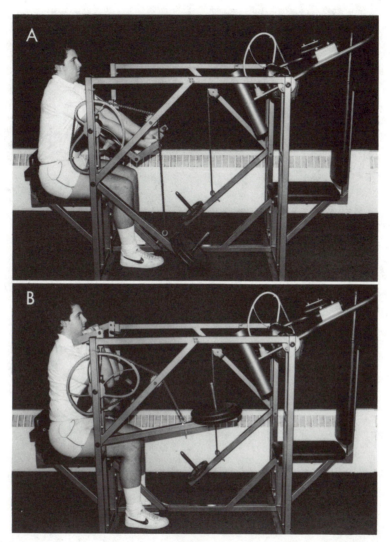

FIG 10–4.
Nautilus biceps/triceps machine. **A,** starting position for the Nautilus biceps curl. Adjust the weight. Sit in the seat and align the elbows with the cams of the machine. Use extra padding if necessary. Keep the back straight. With palms up, grasp the bar with both hands at the curved portion. **B,** full biceps flexion. From the position in **A,** raise the weight by pulling the bar to the chin. Hold this position for 2 seconds, then slowly lower to the count of four, to the starting position. Keep the back straight while doing this exercise. Concentrate on pulling with the arms, not the shoulders and back.

Do ten repetitions of wrist flexion, then ten repetitions of wrist extension, and continue to alternate sets, until completing three sets of ten repetitions for each exercise. Once three sets have been done, rest for five minutes. Then do three more sets of each, once again alternating between extension and flexion. Apply ice for 15 to 20 minutes.

Finally, in sports such as football and wrestling, an adhesive strapping may be useful to provide support during activity.

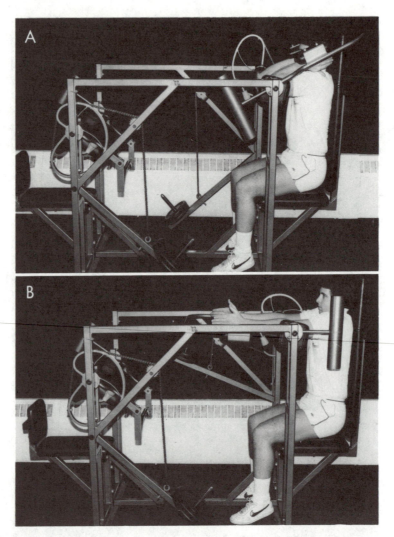

FIG 10–5.
A, the starting position for the triceps extension. Set the appropriate weight. Sit in the seat and place the elbows on the pads in front, aligning them with the cams of the machine. Place the hands behind the pads at the shoulders so that the little fingers touch the pads and the thumbs are toward the shoulders. Adjust the padding so that the elbows are slightly higher than the shoulders. **B,** full triceps extension. From the position in **A,** push against the pads with the hands, moving the elbow through the range of motion until full extension is reached. Hold this position for 2 seconds, then return slowly to the count of four to the starting position. Concentrate on keeping the elbows on the pad. Repeat 8 to 12 times.

INJURY: TENNIS ELBOW

"Tennis elbow" is a general diagnosis that has been used to refer to a variety of injuries. Consequently, this series of injuries has been treated generally, and often inadequately. Pain is the common characteristic for the several different etiologies that can be evaluated.[9] Symptoms include tenderness over the lateral

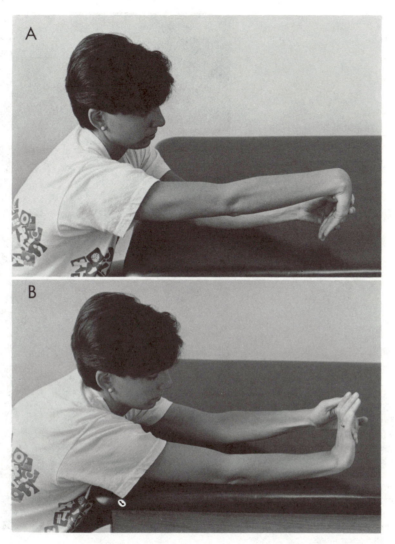

FIG 10–6.
A, wrist flexor stretch. Actively pull the fingers and wrist into the fully flexed position. Flex for 10 seconds, rest. Repeat ten times. **B,** wrist extensor stretch. Actively pull the fingers and wrist into the fully extended position. Extend for 10 seconds. rest. Repeat ten times.

epicondyle, pain with gripping and wrist extension, and limited wrist flexion.[1, 9] Strains or tears of muscle at the tendinous junction can cause pain on palpation of the musculotendinous junction of the extensor carpi radialis brevis muscle. Partial tears of the tendons at their origin and repeated trauma by forceful contraction of the wrist extensors leads to an inflammatory condition, epicondylitis, and the formation of granulation tissue and adhesions.[9] This leads to pain on palpation over the lateral epicondyle. Injury can be exacerbated by forceful contraction of the wrist extensors.[9] Pain at the lateral epicondyle occurs ten times more frequently than at the medial epicondyle.[8]

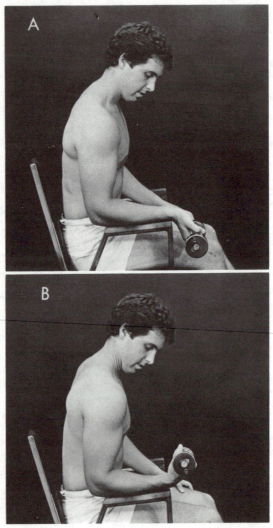

FIG 10–7.
Isotonic strengthening/wrist flexion. **A,** the starting position for the wrist flexion exercise. The elbow is flexed to 90 degrees, the palm is up, and the wrist is fully extended. **B,** the fully flexed position. From the position in **A,** flex the wrist through the range of motion. Hold full flexion for 1 second, then lower slowly to the starting position.

Nirschl subdivides treatment for tennis elbow into four subcategories. The first phase, local conservative treatment for tennis elbow, resembles that for medial epicondylitis. Nirschl advocates cryotherapy and gentle stretching in order to relieve initial inflammation. In acute cases, phenylbutazone or anti-inflammatory agents will reduce inflammation. Cortisone, phenylbutazone, aspirin, and, occasionally, steroids, are other forms of medical treatment.[11–13] Eventually heat can be applied, once inflammation has subsided,[11–13] and ultrasound, whirlpool, and massage are additional adjunctive therapies.[11–13]

Immobilization, in the form of rest with splinting or wrapping with an elastic bandage, can last from three to four days to two weeks, as determined by pain.

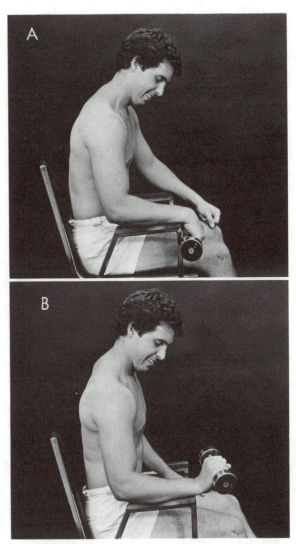

FIG 10–8.
Isotonic strengthening/wrist extension. **A,** the starting position for the wrist extension exercise. The elbow is flexed to 90 degrees, the palm is down, and the wrist is in full flexion. **B,** the fully extended position. From the position in **A,** extend the wrist through the range of motion. Hold full extension for 1 second, then lower slowly to the starting position.

REHABILITATION PROGRAM

For the second phase, Nirschl outlines a rehabilitation program for tennis elbow.[11–13] The aim of the exercises is to improve flexibility and increase strength and endurance. The wrist, forearm, arm, and shoulder are all affected.

Supportive Measures

A forearm band should be used for playing, to reduce sliding of the extensors over the lateral condyle. It acts as an origin for the muscles, and also acts as a reminder to the player[8] (Fig 10–9).

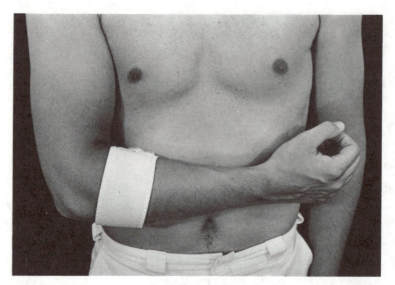

FIG 10–9.
The Nirschl tennis elbow support.

Reduction of Force Loads

The third section of Nirschl's treatment program consists of the reduction of the force loads placed on the forearm extensor group. This can be achieved by changes in technique and alterations in equipment.[11–13]

Surgery

The fourth category is surgical treatment, which is to be used when conservative treatment has not proved effective. Postoperative management should involve the application of a half cast for ten days, and the rehabilitation exercises described below should be performed.[11–13]

REHABILITATION FOR TENNIS ELBOW

The following rehabilitation program is implemented at the University of Pennsylvania Sports Medicine Center. With tennis elbow exercises, emphasis is placed on wrist extension and lateral stretching.

Wrist Flexor Stretch.—Place the palms of the hands together. Raise the elbows upward, pushing the hands together. Hold for 6 to 10 seconds; relax and repeat six to ten times (see Fig 11–1).

Wrist Extensor Stretch.—Place the backs of the hands together. Lower the elbows to the floor, pushing the hands together. Hold for 6 to 10 seconds; relax and repeat six to ten times (see Fig 11–2).

Forearm Flexor Stretching Exercise.—Sit on a stool and rest the arm and elbow, fully extended, on a table. With the opposite hand, actively pull the fingers and wrist into the fully flexed position. Hold for 10 seconds, rest, and repeat. Repeat 10 times (Fig 10–6,A).

Forearm Extensor Stretching Exercise.—Sit on a stool and rest the arm and elbow, fully extended, on a table. With the opposite hand, actively pull the fingers and wrist into the fully extended position. Hold for 10 seconds, rest, and repeat. Repeat 10 times (Fig 10–6,B).

Strengthening

Wrist Flexions.—Place the forearm on a flat surface, palm up. Bend the elbow to 90 degrees. Grasp a dumbbell (weight) and allow it to pull the wrist into the fully extended position. Slowly flex the wrist until it is fully flexed. Hold this position for 1 second then slowly return it to the starting position (see Figs 10–7,A and B).

Wrist Extension.—Place the forearm on a flat surface, palm down. Bend the elbow to 90 degrees. Grasp a dumbbell (weight) and allow it to pull the wrist into the fully flexed position. Slowly extend the wrist until it is fully extended. Hold this position for 1 second then slowly return it to the starting position (see Figs 10–8,A and B).

Repeat three sets of ten repetitions for each of the wrist flexion and extension exercises. Rest five minutes, and then perform three more sets of each. Apply ice to the elbow for 15 to 20 minutes. This exercise program should be repeated once a day. In addition to the above program, the following exercises can also be performed.

Radial Deviation/Ulnar Deviation Exercises.—Place the forearm on a flat surface with the palm down, and rotate the wrist so that the thumb is up. Grasp a dumbbell (weight), and allow it to pull the wrist down into the fully flexed position with radial deviation. Pull up until the wrist is fully extended with radial deviation; hold this position for 1 second, then slowly lower it to the starting position, and continue for three sets of 10 repetitions each (Figs 10–10,A and B).

Broomstick Exercises.—Attach a weight (2.5 lb) to a rope and tie the rope to the middle of a broomstick handle.

1. With palms facing up, flex each wrist one at a time, turning the broomstick handle so that the rope wraps around it and raises the weight. Lower the weight slowly by extending each wrist, one at a time.
2. Repeat the above exercises with the palms facing the floor. Raise the weight by extending each wrist one at a time, and lower it by flexing each wrist. Do 20 repetitions of each, once a day. Begin with a 2.5 lb weight, and gradually progress to 10 lb.[8]

Gripping Exercises.—Use a "Silly Putty" or other therapeutic-type putty. Start with moderate-intensity gripping, squeeze the "putty" for 2 to 3 seconds, and repeat 15 times. Increase intensity of grip to correspond to increased intensity in wrist flexion and wrist extension exercises.

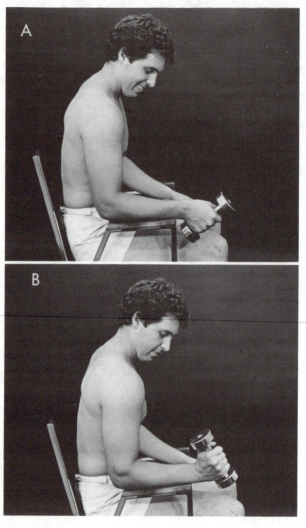

FIG 10–10.
Isotonic strengthening/radial-ulnar deviation. **A,** the starting position for radial-ulnar deviation exercises. The elbow is flexed to 90 degrees, the wrist is rotated so that the thumb is up, and the wrist is in full flexion with radial deviation. **B,** the wrist in full extension with radial deviation. From the position in **A,** extend the wrist through the range of motion. Hold full extension for 1 second, then lower slowly to the starting position.

INJURY: MEDIAL EPICONDYLITIS

The flexor and pronator muscles arise along the medial epicondyle of the humerus. Irritation can develop at the aponeurotic attachment. Epicondylitis is an inflammation of these tissues adjoining the epicondyle of the humerus. Symptoms include pain along the epicondyle, increased pain with gripping, and tenderness localized to the epicondyle or along the supracondylar ridge. The injury is caused by chronic strain and overuse.

Degenerative changes of the connective tissue in combination with overexertion is thought to be a major contributing factor, since most athletes who sustain this injury are middle-aged. Isometric contraction of the forearm is also a contributing factor.[10]

Conservative Treatment

Epicondylitis can be treated conservatively with rest, application of ice, and local injection of corticosteroid if necessary.

Problem: Limited Range of Motion and Weakness

Wrist extension and flexion may be limited in motion and lacking in strength. Stretching and strengthening exercises will be required to alleviate these problems. In addition, strengthening of the flexor-pronator muscles is essential to recovery. This rehabilitation program of local conservative measures and stretching and strengthening exercises is similar to the program advocated for the treatment of lateral epicondylitis, or tennis elbow, by Nirschl.[11–13]

REHABILITATION EXERCISES FOR EPICONDYLITIS

The following rehabilitation program can be performed. Emphasis is placed on wrist flexion and medial stretching.

Stretching
Wrist Flexor Stretch.—Place the palms of the hands together. Raise the elbows upward, pushing the hands together. Hold for 10 seconds; relax and repeat ten times (see Fig 11–1).

Wrist Extensor Stretch.—Place the backs of the hands together. Lower the elbows to the floor, pushing the hands together. Hold for 10 seconds; relax and repeat ten times (see Fig 11–2).

Forearm Extensor and Flexor Stretching Exercises.—Follow the steps given below.

1. Sit on a stool and rest the arm, elbow fully extended, on a table. With the opposite hand, actively pull the fingers and wrist into a fully flexed position. Flex for 10 Seconds, rest. Repeat 10 times (see Fig 10–6,A).
2. Begin as in step 1. With the opposite hand, actively pull the fingers and wrist into the fully extended position. Extend for 10 seconds, rest. Repeat 10 times (see Fig 10–6,B).

Strengthening
Wrist Flexions.—Place the forearm on a flat surface, palm up. Bend the elbow to 90 degrees. Grasp a dumbbell (weight) and allow it to pull the wrist into the fully extended position. Slowly flex the wrist until it is fully flexed. Hold this position for 1 second, then slowly return it to the starting position (see Figs 10–7,A and B).

Wrist Extension.—Place the forearm on a flat surface, palm down. Bend the elbow to 90 degrees. Grasp a dumbbell (weight) and allow it to pull the wrist into the fully flexed position. Slowly extend the wrist until it is fully extended. Hold this position for 1 second then slowly return it to the starting position (see Figs 10–8,A and B).

Radial Deviation/Ulnar Deviation Exercises.—Place the forearm on a flat surface with the palm down, and rotate the wrist so that the thumb is up. Grasp a dumbbell (weight) and allow it to pull the wrist down into the fully flexed position with radial deviation. Pull up until the wrist is fully extended with radial deviation. Hold this position for 1 second, then slowly lower it to the starting position (see Figs 10–10,A and B).

Do ten repetitions of wrist flexion, then ten repetitions of wrist extension, and continue to alternate sets, until you have done three sets of ten repetitions for each exercise. Once three sets of each have been done, rest for five minutes. Then do three more sets of each, once again alternating between extension and flexion.

Place ice on the elbow for 15 to 20 minutes.

This exercise program should be repeated once per day. You should start with 2.5 lb of weight and increase to 10 lbs per week if possible.

Similar exercises can be done with variations in positioning. Wrist extension can be done with radial deviation and ulnar deviation, and pronation, supination, and wrist circles can also be done.[9]

Broomstick Exercises.—Attach a weight (2.5 lb) to a rope and tie the rope to the middle of a broomstick handle.

1. With palms facing up, flex each wrist one at a time, turning the broomstick handle so that the rope wraps around it and raises the weight. Lower the weight slowly by extending each wrist one at a time.
2. Repeat the above exercises with the palms facing the floor, and raise the weight by extending each wrist one at a time, and lower it by flexing each wrist. Do 20 repetitions of each, once a day. Begin with a 2.5 lb weight, and gradually progress to 10 lb.[10]

Gripping Exercises.—Use "Silly Putty" or other therapeutic-type putty. Start with moderate intensity gripping; squeeze the "putty" 2 to 3 seconds and repeat 15 times. Increase intensity of grip to correspond to increased intensity in wrist flexion and wrist extension exercises.

Dynasplint

The Dynasplint is a recently developed spring-tension, low-load, prolonged-stretch device. It is used to increase joint motion that has been reduced by soft tissue contracture following immobilization. The concept of increasing range of motion through prolonged stretching at moderate tension was introduced by Kottke et al.[7] in the 1960s.

The splint is composed of two adjustable cuffs that encircle the upper arm and forearm. The sailcloth cuffs can expand from 6 to 18 in. for the upper arm and 6 to 11 in. for the lower arm. Medial and lateral stabilization bars parallel the long axis of the humerus and the ulna. These stainless steel struts are adjustable from 6½ to 9⅛ in. in five increments for the upper arm and from 7½ to 10½ in. in four increments for the lower arm. The struts articulate by a hinge at the center of the elbow joint axis. A tension spring, housed in each of the two forearm stabilizing bars, is adjustable from 1 lb to 12 lb. The total weight is 1.5 lb (Fig 10–11).[16]

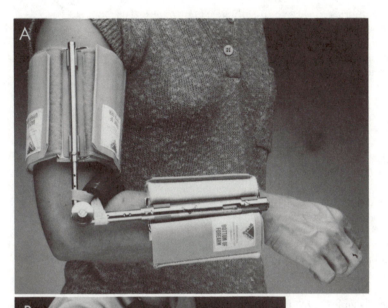

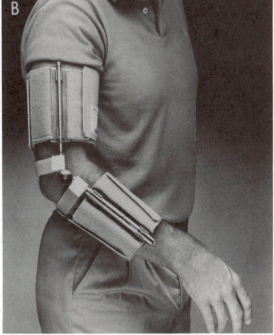

FIG 10–11.
A, the elbow flexion Dynasplint for 50 to 140 degrees of flexion. **B,** the elbow extension Dynasplint for 65 degrees of flexion to 0+ degrees extension.

Both elbow flexion and extension can be increased with the use of Dynasplint (see Figs 10–11,A and B). (Dynasplint is manufactured by Dynasplint Systems, Inc. To order call 1-800-638-6771; for more information contact Dynasplint Systems Inc., 6655 Amberton Drive, Suite A, Baltimore, MD 21227, 301-796-5595.)

REFERENCES

1. Adams JE: Bone injuries in very young athletes. *Clin Orthop* 1968; 58:129.
2. Adams JE: Injury to the throwing arm. A study of traumatic changes in the elbow joint of boy baseball players. *Calif Med* 1965; 102:127.
3. Ellman H: Osteochondrosis of the radial head. Scientific exhibit at the annual meeting of the American Academy of Orthopedic Surgeons. Washington DC, 1972.
4. Grana WA, Rashkin A: Pitcher's elbow in adolescents. *Am J Sports Med* 1980; 8(5):333–336.
5. Indelicato PA, Jobe FW, Kerlan RK, et al: Correctable elbow lesions in professional baseball players: A review of 25 cases. *Am J Sports Med* 1979; 7(1):72–75.
6. Kivi P: The etiology and conservative treatment of humeral epicondylitis. *Scand J Rehab Med* 1982; 15:37–41.
7. Kottke FJ, Pauley DL, Ptak KA: The rationale for prolonged stretching for correction of shortening of connective tissue. *Arch Phys Med Rehabil* 1966; 47:345–352.
8. Kulund DN, McCue FC, Rockwell DA, et al: Tennis injuries: Prevention and treatment. *Am J Sports Med* 1979; 7(4):249–253.
9. LaFreniere JG: 'Tennis elbow': Evaluation, treatment, prevention. *Physical Therapy* 1979; 59:742–746.
10. McCue FC: The elbow, wrist and hand, in Kulund DN (ed): *The Injured Athlete*. Philadelphia JB Lippincott Co, 1982, pp 295–329.
11. Nirschl RP: Defining and treating 'Tennis elbow.' *Contemp Surg* 1977; 10:13–17.
12. Nirschl RP: Tennis elbow. *Orthop Clin North Am* 1973; 4:787–800.
13. Nirschl RP: Tennis elbow. *Primary Care* 1977; 4:367–382.
14. O'Donaghue DH: Injuries of the elbow, in O'Donaghue DH (ed): *The Treatment of Injuries to Athletes*. Philadelphia, WB Saunders Co, 1984, pp 221–246.
15. Pappas AM: Elbow problems associated with baseball during childhood and adolescence. *Clin Orthop* 1982; 164:30–41.
16. Richard RL: Use of the Dynasplint to correct elbow flexion burn contracture: A case report. *J Burn Care Rehabil* 1986; 7:151–152.
17. Torg JS: Little League: 'The theft of a carefree youth.' *Phys Sports Med* 1973; 1:72–78.
18. Tullos HS, King JW: Lesions of the pitching arm in adolescents. *JAMA* 1972; 220:264.
19. Wilson FD, Andrews JR, Blackburn TA, et al: Valgus extension overload in the pitching elbow. *Am J Sports Med* 1983; 11(2):83–88.

CHAPTER 11

The Wrist and Hand

THE WRIST

There are a number of injuries that can occur to the structures in and around the wrist. While sprains are rare, tenosynovitis, tendinitis, nerve entrapment, and fractures are common. This chapter will not cover every variation that can occur, but will discuss prototypical injuries, the mechanism involved, the relevant symptoms, and the treatment and rehabilitation procedures.

INJURY: DE QUERVAIN'S DISEASE

De Quervain's disease is a constrictive tenosynovitis that can afflict the wrist. Overuse of the wrist and thumb can cause swelling of the long abductor and short extensor tendons as they pass through the same sheath of the compartment. Symptoms include pain and swelling over the styloid of the radius. Palpation of the styloid reveals tenderness and firmness.[9]

Treatment for cases that are diagnosed early should consist of immobilization of the thumb and wrist, and injection with a local anesthetic and corticosteroid. In rare instances, de Quervain's disease may require surgical treatment, and this should be followed by immobilization in a splint for two weeks, if not longer. Protection should continue several weeks after the sutures are removed.[9]

REHABILITATION

Following immobilization or after surgery, rehabilitation exercises should be instituted. Stretching and strengthening exercises are effective in restoring range of motion and lost strength. The program of exercises utilized by University of Pennsylvania Sports Medicine Center are described toward the end of this chapter.

INJURY: CARPAL TUNNEL SYNDROME

Carpal tunnel syndrome[9] results from entrapment of the median nerve in the carpal tunnel. This injury may be initiated by direct trauma or by intrusion of a mass into the tunnel area. Surgical findings include swelling of the structures in the volar compartment, as well as constriction of the carpal tunnel. A tingling sensation occurs in the distribution of the median nerve due to pressure on the nerve. Additional symptoms include tenderness, increased pain, and paresthesia with deep pressure on the volar ligament.[9] Immobilization can be an effective treatment when the injury is diagnosed early. It helps to rest the swollen parts, decrease inflammation, and prevent the tendon from sliding over the nerve.[9] If conservative treatment is not effective then the injury can be treated surgically, followed by immobilization in a forearm splint for two to three weeks. Free movement of the fingers should be allowed after the first 48 hours.[9] Again, immobilization should be followed by rehabilitation exercises described at the end of this chapter.

INJURY: FRACTURES

There are a variety of different fractures that can occur in the wrist area. Among them are carpal navicular, hamate, hamate hook, lunate, and fractures of the radius and ulna (Colles' fractures). The three prototypical fractures to be discussed here are navicular, Bennett's, and Colles' fractures.

Fractures of the carpal navicular bone are the most common wrist fractures that occur in athletes. The navicular has an anatomical predisposition to injury. It is usually injured as a result of forced hyperextension, such as a fall on an outstretched hand.[7] Symptoms include pain and swelling through the wrist and localized pain between the thumb and the distal end of the radius at the anatomical "snuffbox." Gripping can be painful. Early diagnosis is important.[7]

Bennett's fractures[3] are fracture dislocations. The carpometacarpal joint of the thumb is disrupted by the fracture line, which usually occurs between the major part of the metacarpal and a volar lip fragment. Axial blows against a partially flexed metacarpal usually cause Bennett's fractures.[2]

Colles' fractures are fractures of the distal radius with posterior displacement. Usually they result from a fall on an outstretched hand.[2] Colles' fractures include extra-articular or intra-articular fractures involving the radiocarpal joint,[2] intra-articular fractures involving the distal radial joint, and the intra-articular fractures involving both radiocarpal and distal radioulnar joints. Symptoms include pain, swelling, weakness, a visible deformity of the wrist, crepitus, limitation of finger motion, numbness, and tenderness with palpation and manipulation.[2]

All three of the above injuries can be treated with immobilization, followed by rehabilitation. Variations in forms and length of immobilization are as follows.

The treatment of choice for undisplaced navicular fractures is immobilized for six to eight weeks in a long-arm thumb spica cast with the wrist in slight radial deviation.[2]

Closed reduction and immobilization of a Bennet's fracture should be attempted. If this is not successful, open reduction followed by immobilization is necessary. Immobilization can consist of a plaster thumb spica cast for four to six weeks.[3]

Most Colles' fractures can best be managed with closed reduction, and immobilization in a long arm cast. The forearm can be placed in either pronation or supination, and the wrist in slight flexion and ulnar deviation. Occasionally, pin and plaster, or external fixation/immobilization is necessary. Reduction of the fracture should be followed by measures to reduce swelling. The arm should be elevated for 48 hours, and finger and shoulder exercises should be performed when the patient has recuperated from anesthesia. These should consist of full excursion of the fingers for a count of 2 seconds. The fingers should be fully extended then fully flexed, at least ten times every half hour. Reapplication of plaster casting might be necessary after about two weeks due to a decrease of swelling. Early adequate reduction of these injuries is important in preventing complications.[2] Again, immobilization should be followed by rehabilitation.

INJURY: GANGLION

Ganglions of the extensor tendon(s) of the wrist occur infrequently in athletes. Two possible causes are cited: (1) degenerative changes in the tendon and (2) synovial herniation. Characteristically there occurs a soft fluctuant mass distal to the dorsal carpal ligament, usually located over the capitate, along with pain during wrist flexion.[9]

Treatment is usually directed at relieving the symptoms by aspiration of the ganglionic contents. If symptoms persist or interfere with normal function, surgical excision of the ganglion may be performed.

REHABILITATION

The principle of regaining motion before attempting to increase strength, as emphasized in the discussions of other areas of the body, applies to the rehabilitation of the wrist. The program implemented by the University of Pennsylvania Sports Medicine Center for rehabilitating the prototypical injuries to the wrist is as follows.

Range of Motion

Range of motion can be improved by stretching the wrist in the following manner.

Wrist Flexor Stretch.—Place the palms of the hands together. Raise the elbows upward, pushing the hands together. Hold this position for 10 seconds. Relax, then repeat ten times (Fig 11–1).

Wrist Extensor Stretch.—Place the backs of the hands together. Lower the elbows while pushing the hands together. Hold this position for 10 seconds. Relax, then repeat ten times (Fig 11–2).

Active Pronation/Supination Stretch.—With the elbow flexed to 90 degrees, rotate the forearm so that the palm faces upward. Hold this position for 10 seconds. Then rotate the arm so that the palm faces down; again, hold for 10 seconds. Continue to rotate back and forth between the two positions, repeating each stretched position ten times.

Active-Assisted Pronation.—Hold a broomstick in the right hand with the palm facing down. Apply downward pressure on the end of the broomstick with the opposite hand so that the wrist rotates into pronation. Hold this position for 10 seconds. Relax, then repeat ten times (Fig 11–3).

Active-Assisted Supination.—Hold the broomstick in the right hand again, this time with the palm up. Apply upward pressure with the opposite hand so that the wrist rotates into full supination. Hold this position for 10 seconds. Relax, then repeat ten times (Fig 11–4).

Radial/Ulnar Deviation Stretch.—With the elbow flexed to 90 degrees, rest the forearm on a table so that the wrist is at the edge. Make a fist and rotate the forearm so that the thumb faces the ceiling. Flex the wrist and hold the stretched position for 10 seconds. Relax and repeat ten times. Then extend the wrist as far as possible, and hold the stretched position for 10 seconds. Relax, then repeat ten times.

FIG 11–1.
Wrist flexion. The fully stretched position for wrist flexion.

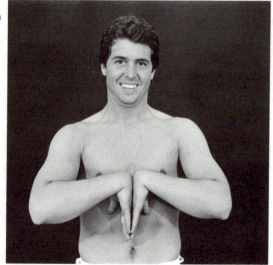

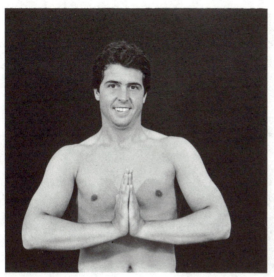

FIG 11–2.
Wrist extension. The fully stretched position for wrist extension.

Strengthening

Strengthening exercises for the wrist include wrist extension and flexion exercises (weights or broomstick), both in a neutral position, and in various alternate positions. Supination and pronation exercises should also be done. Grip strength exercises are also effective. These exercises should be performed as follows.

Wrist Flexion.—Place the forearm on a flat surface, palm up. Bend the elbow to 90 degrees. Grasp a dumbbell (weight) and allow it to pull the wrist into the fully extended position. Slowly flex the wrist until it is fully flexed. Hold this position for 1 second, and then slowly return it to the starting position (see Figs 10–7,A and B).

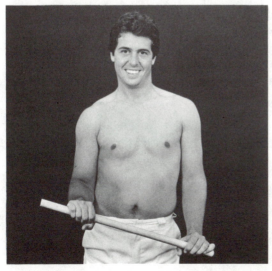

FIG 11–3.
Pronation. Active-assisted pronation of the right wrist, using the broomstick. The palm is facing down, and downward pressure with the left hand is being applied on the broomstick, causing the wrist to rotate into pronation.

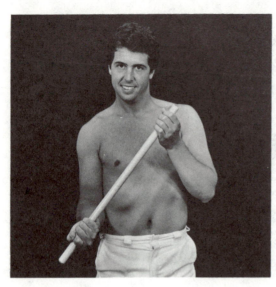

FIG 11–4.
Supination. With the palm up, the wrist is rotated into full supination by applying upward pressure to the broomstick with the opposite hand.

Wrist Extension.—Place the forearm on a flat surface, palm down. Bend the elbow to 90 degrees. Grasp a dumbbell (weight) and allow it to pull the wrist into the fully flexed position. Slowly extend the wrist until it is fully extended. Hold this position for 1 second, then slowly return it to the starting position (see Figs 10–8,A and B).

Do ten repetitions of wrist flexion, then ten repetitions of wrist extension, and continue to alternate sets until completing three sets of ten repetitions for each exercise. Once three sets have been done, rest for five minutes. Then do three more sets of each, once again alternating between extension and flexion.

Place ice on the wrist for 15 to 20 minutes.

This exercise should be repeated once a day. Start with 2.5 lb of weight and increase to 10 lb.

Similar exercises can be done with variations in positioning. Wrist extension can be done with radial deviation and ulnar deviation, pronation, supination, and broomstick can also be performed.[5]

Radial Deviation/Ulnar Deviation Exercises.—Place the forearm on a flat surface with the palm down, and rotate the wrist so that the thumb is up. Grasp a dumbbell (weight) and allow it to pull the wrist down into the fully flexed position with radial deviation. Pull up until the wrist is fully extended with radial deviation, hold this position for 1 second, then slowly lower it to the starting position, and continue back and forth for one minute (see Figs 10–10,A and B).

Pronation/Supination Exercises.—Perform the pronation/supination exercises described above under active-assisted stretching, except give resistance with the right arm as the pressure is applied by the left.

Broomstick Exercises.—Attach a weight (2.5 lb) to a rope and tie the rope to the middle of the broomstick handle.

1. With palms facing up, flex each wrist (one at a time), turning the broomstick handle so that the rope wraps around it and raises the weight. Lower the weight slowly by extending each wrist (one at a time).
2. Repeat the above exercise with the palms facing the floor, and raise the weight by extending each wrist (one at a time), and lower it by flexing each wrist. Do 20 repetitions of each. Begin with a 2.5 lb weight, and gradually progress to 10 lb.[4]

HAND INJURIES

MALLET FINGER

Mallet finger, an extensor mechanism injury, can result from flexion or hyperflexion against resistance. This causes the extensor tendon to rupture from its insertion.[6] Distal interphalangeal joint extensor mechanism injuries result in inability of the athlete to extend the terminal phalanx.

Treatment

In cases in which the bone fragment has not been avulsed, treatment usually involves splinting the distal interphalangeal joint in full hyperextension and the proximal interphalangeal joint in 90 degrees of flexion. Surgical reduction of the avulsed fragment may be necessary. Athletic participation may continue if the finger is splinted. This form of support should be maintained for six to eight weeks. This injury is common in athletic activities that involve catching.[6]

INJURY: GAMEKEEPER'S THUMB

An injury to the thumb referred to as gamekeeper's thumb[6] results when the ulnar collateral ligament is torn from its attachment to the proximal phalanx.[6] This results in instability and interferes with pinch.

Closed treatment can be used for partial tears, and open repair and reduction for complete. Surgical repair should be followed by immobilization in a splint or thumb spica cast for five weeks. When the athlete returns to activity, the thumb should be taped to prevent abduction.

METACARPAL FRACTURE

Fractures at the base of the metacarpal are characterized by extreme tenderness and pain with direct pressure over the injured area.[6] A direct blow at the end of the shaft can cause this fracture.

Reduction can be attempted via traction. If this fails, internal fixation may be necessary. Fractures in the shaft usually resolve with mobilization. Internal fixation is sometimes necessary and is required more often in oblique rather than transverse fractures. Traction and reduction can be followed by the use of a volar splint, with the wrist in dorsiflexion, the metacarpophalangeal joint semi-flexed, and proximal interphalangeal joint sharply flexed to 90 degrees, with a pressure pad adjacent to the fracture sight.

Fractures to the neck of the metacarpal occur quite often. Reduction of these fractures is more readily attained than some others. Splinting the finger while the proximal phalanx is flexed to 90 degrees is thought to provide greater stability. Kulund's experience with this is not favorable. He recommends internal fixation with K-wire.[6]

PHALANGES

Fractures and dislocation of the phalanges occur frequently in athletes. These should not be managed in a cavalier fashion; all finger injuries should be x-rayed and appropriate treatment instituted by a qualified physician. Care should be taken to manage these injuries in the same manner as one would manage a similar injury in a nonathlete. Importance should be placed on returning the finger and hand to normal function.

BOUTONNIÈRE DEFORMITY

Boutonnière deformity involves an avulsion of the central extensor tendon slip at the proximal interphalangeal joint. It is characterized by an inability to actively extend the proximal interphalangeal joint. Delay in treatment can result in a flexion contracture, which must be treated with splinting.

Treatment for the different fractures in the hand is basically the same, with certain variations. Essentially it consists of reducing the fracture dislocation with traction, pressure, and immobilization. Immobilization positioning will vary for different injuries. If accurate reduction cannot be obtained or maintained then internal fixation will be necessary. Surgery should be followed by immobilization and appropriate rehabilitation.[6]

REHABILITATION

Rehabilitation of hand injuries can be complicated and may require the supervision of an occupational therapist. For nonoperative problems we concentrate on range of motion and strength and recommend gripping exercises, with either gripping putty or a tennis ball. In addition to gripping exercises, pinching both small and large objects will help rehabilitate the injury. In the case of hand rehabilitation, it is important that symmetrical range of motion be maintained.

Gripping Exercises

Use a tennis ball or other gripping-type device. Start with moderate-intensity gripping, which is held for 2 to 3 seconds, and repeat 15 times. Increase intensity of grip to correspond to increase intensity in wrist flexion and wrist extension exercises.

REFERENCES

1. Beckenbaugh RD: Accurate evaluation and management of the painful wrist following injury. *Orthop Clin North Am* 1984; 15:289–306.
2. Dobyns JH, Linscheid RL: Fractures and dislocations of the wrist, in Rockwood CA, Green DP (eds): *Fractures*. Philadelphia, JB Lippincott Co, 1975, vol 1, pp 345–440.
3. Green DP, Rowland SA: Fractures and dislocations in the hand, in Rockwood CA, Green DP (eds): *Fractures*. Philadelphia, JB Lippincott Co, 1975, vol 1, pp 265–343.
4. Kulund DN, McCue FC, Rockwell DA, et al: Tennis injuries: Prevention and treatment: A review. *Am J Sports Med* 1979; 7:249–253.
5. LaFreniere JG: 'Tennis elbow': evaluation, treatment, prevention. *Physical Therapy* 1979; 59:742–746.
6. McCue C: Elbow, wrist, and hand, in Kulund DN (ed): *The Injured Athlete.* Philadelphia, JB Lippincott Co, 1982, pp 295–329.
7. McCue FC, Baugher WH, Kulund DN, et al: Hand and wrist injuries in the athlete. *Am J Sports Med* 1979; 7(5):275–286.
8. O'Brien ET: Acute fractures and dislocations of the carpus. *Orthop Clin North Am* 1984; 15:237–258.
9. O'Donaghue DH: Injuries of the wrist, in O'Donaghue DH (ed): *Treatment of Injuries to Athletes.* Philadelphia, WB Saunders Co, 1984, pp 256–285.

CHAPTER 12

Athletic Injuries and the Use of Medication

Neta A. Hodge, Pharm.D.

Clinical Pharmacist, Philadelphia, Pennsylvania

ANALGESIA IN SPORTS RELATED INJURIES

Sports injuries vary widely from mild to severe, but common to most is pain. Pain acts as an integral component of the body's defense system to alert an athlete that an injury or trauma has occurred, so that the affected area can be protected from further injury. Regardless of the type of injury causing it, pain can be classified as mild, moderate, or severe; it is a universal symptom, but a highly personal experience.

Several classes of analgesic drugs are available to treat pain. The choice of which agent to use depends on the severity of the pain and individual patient variables, such as drug allergies or concomitant disease states. The spectrum of analgesics available ranges from nonprescription drugs to opiates; proper characterization of the pain via patient interview can guide the clinician in the choice of appropriate analgesic therapy.

Cryotherapy

Immediately following an acute sports injury, the affected area should be immobilized and elevated, and ice should be applied. Ice may be applied in many forms, but rapid application is important. For example, an ice bath, ice massage, or an ice pack can be used. Ski patrols commonly use snow in a plastic bag, applied before the injured skier is transported from the slopes. When ice is applied to the traumatized area and tissue cooling occurs, several physiological responses ensue: Vasoconstriction results and decreases inflammation, edema and blood leakage. Impulses via cooled nerve fibers are slowed, and pain is decreased. Local tissue metabolism is slowed so that oxygen needs and histamine release are decreased. Monosynaptic stretch reflexes are suppressed and muscle spasm is retarded.[17, 37]

Ice should be applied to the affected area for 15 to 20 minutes several times per day. Although a feeling of cold and aching or burning may occur for the first one to seven minutes after the application of ice, a local anesthetic action is to be expected within 5 to 12 minutes after ice is applied.[17] While some studies have demonstrated a reflex vasodilation after the local anesthetic effect occurs, other studies have not corroborated this; this point remains an area of controversy.[14, 17] Hocutt et al.[17] demonstrated that the use of immobilization, compression by use of taping, elevation, and ice (e.g., cryotherapy), when applied within 36 hours of the occurrence of grade 3 or 4 ankle sprains, was more effective than either cryotherapy initiated more than 36 hours after the injury or the application of heat therapy within 36 hours of the injury. Patients receiving cryotherapy within 36 hours of the injury regained full activity in 13.2 days, while those patients on heat therapy required 33.3 days. Those on cryotherapy instituted after 36 hours required 30.4 days to regain full activity.

Cautions associated with the use of ice include avoidance of local frostbite by limiting direct ice application to the skin to periods of less than 30 minutes, and avoidance of the use of ice in any patient who has cold allergy, rheumatoid arthritis, peripheral vascular disease, or other vasoactive disorders such as Raynaud's phenomenon.[17]

Nonopiate Analgesics

Although cryotherapy is commonly the initial therapy in most acute sports injuries, additional pharmacologic analgesia is usually necessary. Several nonprescription analgesics are available to treat mild to moderate pain; these include acetaminophen, salicylates, and ibuprofen.

Acetaminophen

On a milligram-to-milligram basis, acetaminophen is equal to aspirin as an analgesic and antipyretic. The mechanism of action of acetaminophen for analgesia is unknown. It is a very weak anti-inflammatory agent, and because of this would be considered a weaker choice than aspirin for treating the posttraumatic pain and inflammation of sports injuries. It is not toxic to the gastrointestinal (GI) tract and does not affect platelet aggregation, so that it may have increased merit in patients with a history of peptic ulcer disease or in those with platelet disorders, closed head injuries, or injury-incurred hematomas. The maximum recommended nonprescription adult daily dose of acetaminophen is 4 gm in divided doses. Increasing individual doses of aspirin or acetaminophen above 650 to 1,000 mg per dose does not increase the analgesic effect of these drugs; a ceiling analgesic effect occurs.[24] Intentional or inadvertent overdosage of acetaminophen can be potentially lethal if the antidote (N-acetylcysteine) is not administered in time and hepatic necrosis results. Hepatotoxic effects are more likely to develop in alcoholics after an overdose than in nondrinking adults. Children under the age of 10 to 12 years are generally the least likely to develop hepatoxicity following an overdose.

Aspirin

Although several salicylate products are available, aspirin will be discussed here as the prototype salicylate. Aspirin is an analgesic, antipyretic, and anti-inflammatory agent. Its mechanism of action, while not completely understood, is thought to be due to blockade of the enzyme cyclo-oxygenase, which oxygenates arachidonic acid to produce prostaglandins. Prostaglandins are produced on a homeostatic basis in most cells of the body, and are necessary for the normal physiologic functioning of most major organs. When trauma occurs, such as in acute sports injuries, prostaglandin production increases on demand at the site of injury, and is thought to help mediate inflammation. Aspirin and the nonsteroidal anti-inflammatory drugs help to decrease edema, pain, and other signs of inflammation by blocking prostaglandin production. Low-dose aspirin (i.e., less than 3 gm/day) is analgesic, but higher doses are anti-inflammatory. High individual variation can occur in patients' responses to aspirin because elimination is nonlinear and accumulation of blood salicylate levels can occur. Because of this it is difficult to declare a specific daily dose of aspirin for everyone; generally, anti-inflammatory doses are considered to range from 3 to 8 gm/day in divided doses. Because aspirin is available so readily without a prescription, many patients may be resistant to taking it and may ask for a "real" pain killer. Aspirin plus cryotherapy provides excellent analgesia for mild to moderate pain with inflammation, such as may occur with mild sprains or strains; patients need to be educated as to aspirin's anti-inflammatory capabilities.

The side effect profile of aspirin can be extensive and side effects or certain individual patient variables may preclude its use. Gastrointestinal effects such as gastritis, ulceration, or hemorrhage can occur, especially at high doses, and its use should be avoided in patients with a history of peptic ulcer disease or a GI tract hemorrhage. Aspirin, by blocking cyclo-oxygenase, inhibits platelet aggregation irreversibly for the life of the platelet. This effect may be of little consequence in most healthy athletes, but those with platelet disorders or bleeding diatheses should avoid its use. The antiplatelet effect of aspirin may be particularly dangerous in those athletes who have sustained an intra-articular hemorrhage or muscular hematoma or a closed head injury. The use of aspirin after these types of injuries is contraindicated because of the danger of further bleeding.

Allergy to aspirin, called "aspirin intolerance," may appear within hours of ingesting the drug, and may take one of two forms: bronchospasm or urticaria-angioedema. Aspirin intolerance, not to be confused with GI upset due to aspirin, is more likely to occur in patients with a history of chronic urticaria, asthma, or chronic rhinitis. It may have a familial pattern and many aspirin intolerant patients are also allergic to tartrazine dye. Antibodies against aspirin have not been demonstrated, but prostaglandin inhibition has been implicated in the mechanism of the bronchospastic form of aspirin intolerance.[30, 35] The use of aspirin and related drugs, such as the nonsteroidal anti-inflammatory drugs, is strictly contraindicated in patients with a history of aspirin intolerance. It is exceedingly important to question patients regarding this before prescribing these drugs, as aspirin intolerance, when it occurs, can be life-threatening.

Aspirin intoxication can occur during short courses of aspirin and at doses considered to be "therapeutic." Because of aspirin's nonlinear elimination, small increases in dosage may result in disproportionate rises in serum salicylate levels. Therapeutic salicylate levels are considered to range from 20 to 30 mg/dl but some patients may exhibit symptoms of intoxication, such as tinnitus or nausea, at dosage and blood levels considered to be "therapeutic." Individualization of the dose, with the use of serum salicylate levels, may alleviate these problems and can allow anti-inflammatory therapy to continue. When given chronically, in anti-inflammatory doses, every 8- or 12-hour doses of aspirin can maintain therapeutic salicylate levels.[23]

Acetaminophen or Aspirin in Combination With Opiate Drugs

Combining aspirin or acetaminophen with opiate analgesics causes an additive increase in the amount of analgesia available with each dose.[3] Depending on the opiate used, the combination of these drugs extends the spectrum of pain to be treated to that of moderate to moderately severe pain. The increase in analgesia may be offset, however, by the side effects of the opiates. These combinations are indicated for short-term management of acute pain.

Nonsteroidal Anti-inflammatory Drugs

The nonsteroidal anti-inflammatory drugs are as effective as aspirin as antipyretic and anti-inflammatory agents. Several of these drugs have been shown to be more effective analgesics than aspirin alone, acetaminophen alone, or either aspirin or acetaminophen in combination with codeine in several pain models.[5, 8] Some nonsteroidal anti-inflammatory drugs have been shown to be equally efficacious to oral and injectable opiates in dental, postoperative, postepisiotomy, and cancer pain models.[36] Only some of the nonsteroidal anti-inflammatory drugs currently available in the United States are approved by the FDA to treat pain. Table 12–1 lists these agents and their recommended doses. Although many health care professionals believe that the nonsteroidal anti-inflammatory drugs are weak analgesics, these drugs have been shown to control moderate to moderately severe pain in many situations. They have the advantage over acetaminophen in that they are anti-inflammatory, over aspirin in that they are stronger analgesics, and over the opiates because they do not cause physical dependence.

Although their exact mechanism of action is unknown, the nonsteroidal anti-inflammatory drugs, like aspirin, are believed to work by means of inhibiting prostaglandin production, thereby blocking the prostaglandins' effects on inflammation. The use of nonsteroidal anti-inflammatory drugs in treating sports-related injuries is increasing, although studies of the use of these drugs in acute sports-related injuries have reported varying results and have been plagued with flaws in study design; very few studies have been double-blinded or placebo-controlled, and some drugs have been studied at suboptimal dosages.[1, 25, 29] Despite this, the nonsteroidal anti-inflammatory drugs are a rational

TABLE 12–1.

Nonsteroidal Anti-inflammatory Drugs Approved by the FDA
for the Treatment of Pain

GENERIC NAME	TRADE NAME	STARTING ADULT DOSE, MG	MAXIMUM RECOMMENDED DOSE, MG
Ibuprofen	Motrin, Rufen	400, 4 times daily	3,200
Nonprescription ibuprofen	Various brands	200, every 4–6 hr	1,200
Naproxen	Naprosyn	500, initially; 250, every 6–8 hr	1,250
Naproxen sodium	Anaprox	550, initially; 275, every 6–8 hr	1,375
Diflunisal	Dolobid	1,000, initially; 500, every 8–12 hr	1,500
Fenoprofen	Nalfon	200, every 4–6 hr	3,200
Mefenamic acid	Ponstel	500, initially; 250, every 6 hr	250, every 6 hr
Suprofen	Suprol	200, every 4–6 hr	800 per day

choice for both analgesic and anti-inflammatory effects in acute and chronic
sports-related injuries and have been reported to permit a faster recovery by
patients.[12] These drugs have side effects, though, and these must be borne in
mind during patient selection for this therapy. The nonsteroidal anti-inflammatory drugs can cause GI toxicity (i.e., ulceration and/or hemorrhage) and although this occurs less frequently than with aspirin, the use of these drugs in
patients with a history of peptic ulcer disease or GI tract bleeding is contraindicated. Platelet aggregation can be affected by the nonsteroidal anti-inflammatory drugs, but this effect is reversible upon discontinuation of the drug. Nev-
ertheless, the use of these drugs in patients with preexistent platelet disorders,
bleeding diatheses, or with hematomas or closed head injuries should be ap-
proached with extreme caution. Patients with aspirin intolerance may have a
greater than 90% probability of cross-reacting when given nonsteroidal anti-
inflammatory drugs,[30] constituting a strict contraindication to the use of these
drugs in this patient group. All of the nonsteroidal anti-inflammatory drugs are
more expensive than aspirin and this may limit their use in some patients. It
has been shown in hospitalized patients that the nonsteroidal anti-inflammatory agents are more economical to use in patients with moderate pain than
the aspirin or acetaminophen combinations with opiates. DEA-controlled sub-
stances must be handled more, with increased paperwork, resulting in hidden
labor costs that increase the cost of the DEA-controlled drugs significantly.[28]
The nonsteroidal anti-inflammatory drugs have been reported to produce acute
renal failure and concomitant electrolyte disturbances in patients with chronic
renal insufficiency, congestive heart failure, systemic lupus erythematosus, cir-
rhosis with ascites, and fluid depletion states. This effect is thought to be a
result of renal prostaglandin inhibition and may be of concern in athletes with
fluid depletion or renal disease. Other side effects of the nonsteroidal anti-inflammatory agents may include central nervous system effects (e.g., headache,
sedation), and rashes.

Opiate Analgesics

Opiate analgesics are indicated for severe pain such as may occur with a fracture, a severe sprain, or after surgery. The term "narcotics" has been supplanted, since the discovery of the opiate receptor, with the more specific term "opiate agonist" to specify the action of this group of drugs at the receptor site. These drugs produce analgesia by competitively binding opiate receptors. Although the main pharmacological action of the opiate agonists is analgesia, these drugs have many other effects throughout the body. Actions in the central nervous system include sedation, mental clouding, mood variations, nausea, vomiting, euphoria, and respiratory depression. The use of opiate agonists in patients with closed head injuries should be avoided so that mental status changes are not masked by the drugs. Release of pituitary hormones such as thyrotropin and luteinizing hormone may be suppressed, while the release of prolactin and growth hormone may be enhanced by the chronic use of opiates. The opiate agonists can cause miosis and also depress the cough reflex. Since a large number of opiate receptors are found in the gastrointestinal tract as well as in the central nervous system, it is not surprising that the opiate agonists cause constipation; effects in the biliary tract may include increased pressure. The clinical effects of the opiate agonists on the smooth muscles of the ureter and the sphincter of the urinary bladder can be especially troublesome and somewhat frightening to the recumbent postoperative patient who experiences difficulty in voiding urine. Hypotension may occur in the nonrecumbent patient due to the release of histamine and the α-adrenergic effects of the opiate agonists. Many opiate agonists are available in oral and parenteral form. The route of administration of opiate agonists affects the dose; oral administration requires higher doses than parenteral administration because significant first-pass metabolism occurs in the liver with oral doses. Duration of action of these drugs is also affected by the route of administration, so that oral dosing generally increases the duration of action by at least one hour.[13] Opiate agonists can cause tolerance, physical and psychological dependence, and a withdrawal syndrome; these side effects may limit the long-term use of opiates in non-cancer patients. The effects of opiate agonists are blocked by opiate antagonists. Mixed opiate agonist-antagonist drugs are also effective in treating pain, but they can cause psychomimetic effects such as hallucinations, and may precipitate a withdrawal syndrome in patients who are physically dependent upon opiate agonist drugs.

The long-term use of opiates in managing pain in the recovering and rehabilitating athlete is not routinely recommended, except in special circumstances, because of the potential for addiction. Anti-inflammatory doses of aspirin or the nonsteroidal anti-inflammatory drugs should suffice in this situation.

CENTRALLY ACTING ORAL MUSCLE RELAXANTS

Many sports-related sprains, strains, and pains have attendant muscle spasms that, if easily alleviated, could allow faster rehabilitation of the affected area. The use of centrally acting oral muscle relaxants would seem rational in this situation; indeed, widespread use of these drugs does occur. But solid evidence for the efficacy of this class of drugs is lacking and controversial. Elenbaas,[11] in an excellent review on this subject, found that it was "not possible to substantiate clearly the superiority of any of the muscle relaxants over an analgesic or sedative, in either acute or chronic conditions," or over other muscle relaxants. Concurrent physical therapy confounds the issue, as its influence on the response of patients (and thus its measured contribution to study results) who are concurrently taking muscle relaxant drugs has not been established. Combination muscle relaxant products seem to relieve pain symptoms better than single-agent products, but comparison of the combination products against the combined use of a sedative and an analgesic has not been done. Clinicians' and patients' beliefs that the centrally acting oral muscle relaxants contribute to recovery will cause a continuation of the use of these agents, but the actual efficacy and role of these drugs in managing muscle spasms will only become clear after appropriate, well-designed, and well-controlled clinical trials provide much-needed proof.

MAINTAINING ELECTROLYTE BALANCE IN ATHLETES

Strenuous exercise, especially in extreme heat and high humidity can result in significant losses of body water via sweat in the athlete. Electrolytes are lost in smaller amounts than water but both the lost fluid and electrolytes must be replaced, or heat disorders may ensue. Deaths in young healthy athletes, although uncommon, have prompted research into the etiology and prevention of heat disorders.

One quart of sweat corresponds to approximately 2 lb of weight loss in the athlete and contains 0.7 to 1.1 gm of sodium in a conditioned, acclimated athlete. The untrained athlete can potentially lose more sodium per quart of sweat (0.5 to 1.8 gm).[38]

For every 100 kcal of energy used in the exercising muscle, 75 to 80 kcal is dissipated as heat waste.[33] The bloodstream carries the heat from the muscle to the lung for partial excretion, to the brain to trigger thermal receptors, and to the skin for dissipation. The skin loses heat by means of radiation to the air, convection, and the evaporation of sweat. The production and evaporation of sweat depends upon adequate body water (e.g., adequate intravascular and extracellular fluid volumes), the intensity of exercise, and the temperature and humidity of the ambient air.

Several heat disorders can occur when excessive amounts of body water and electrolytes are lost via single episodes of intensive exercise, or, more commonly, in accumulated losses over a period of days due to inadequate replacement. Heat cramps, most common in the gastrocnemius or hamstring muscles, are caused by water depletion, not salt loss, and are easily prevented by adequate water intake during exercise. Heat syncope and its attendant weakness are easily treated with water and rest. Heat exhaustion, also called heat collapse, is caused by a depletion of the intravascular fluid volume. Its symptoms range from dizziness, headache, vomiting, and weakness, to loss of consciousness.

Profuse sweating and normal or slight body temperature increases are seen. Fluid loss must be repleted, the athlete must rest, and evaluation of the athlete's fluid status must be done before he or she resumes exercise. Heat stroke is life-threatening; it is a result of massive water depletion and may occur in the absence of the previously described heat disorders. It occurs because the body's normal heat regulating systems cannot continue to function in the face of massive fluid deficits. Coma, shock, lack of sweating, and very high core body temperatures ensue. The athlete's body must be cooled immediately, usually by the total-body application of ice or ice water; if quick cooling does not occur, damage to the brain, liver, or kidney, coagulopathies, and/or death may result. Immediate transport to a hospital is mandatory, as heat stroke is a medical emergency.[26]

Prevention is the key to managing heat disorders. Education of athletes and coaches is essential, so that particular attention is paid to heat, humidity, the amount of clothing worn, and weight loss of athletes; copious amounts of ice water must be available and consumed by exercising athletes. Although heat disorders can occur in any athlete, those groups identified at particular risk are preadolescent athletes with a history of heat disorders or a recent febrile illness, unconditioned obese athletes training for high school football teams, and distance runners.[33]

The use of oral electrolyte solutions to replace electrolyte loss has become controversial, and as such, is becoming less common. Liberal salting at meals can replace 8 to 12 gm of sodium per day.[38] Thus, adequate water intake and a well-balanced diet appear adequate to replace fluid and electrolyte deficits in most athletes. Research has shown that oral potassium supplementation can actually increase the urinary loss of potassium and sodium in conditioned long-distance runners during hot, humid weather.[22] Salt tablets should not be used to replace sodium.

MANAGING ASTHMA IN THE ATHLETE

Exercise can induce bronchospasm in a small minority of normal athletes and in most athletes with asthma. Immediately after exercise is begun in these athletes, mild bronchodilation occurs; if exercise is continued, bronchoconstriction can follow within two to ten minutes and will worsen for several minutes after exercise is stopped.[2, 7, 15, 31] Symptoms of coughing, wheezing, or shortness of breath will resolve over the next 30 to 90 minutes,[7] and for the following three to four hours the subject will be refractory to another attack.[15] A small percentage of athletes may experience a reaction as late as three to eight hours after exercise.[4] The cause of exercise-induced asthma is unknown, but two hypotheses are currently under intense investigation. The first, the respiratory heat loss hypothesis, states that a fall in pulmonary airway temperature, caused by hyperventilation of unwarmed and unhumidified air into the lower airways, results in mucosal temperature changes; this causes decreases in temperatures within the intrathoracic airways, and results in bronchospasm. The respiratory water loss hypothesis states that water loss during humidification of unconditioned air in the airways leads to hyperosmolarity in the airway mucosa, with the resultant occurrence of bronchospasm.[15] Regardless of the mechanism, attacks of exercise-induced asthma can be prevented in most athletes by the inhalation of β_2-sympathomimetic agonists prior to exercise. Albuterol has been reported as having superiority in this regard because of its extended duration of action.[32] Theophylline and cromolyn sodium used prophylactically can also help to prevent exercise-induced asthma attacks to a lesser degree than aerosolized β_2-agonists (particularly albuterol).[20] Calcium-channel blocking drugs show some promise in preventing exercise-induced asthma. Underlying asthma in the athlete should be stabilized with theophylline given at regular doses, if necessary, to increase the likelihood of the prophylaxis of attacks being successful with inhaled drugs. The International Olympic Committee allows the use of oral theophylline, inhaled glucocorticosteroids, inhaled cromolyn sodium, and the β_2-agonists, terbutaline or albuterol, by asthmatic athletes in international competition. Doses of these drugs may vary widely because of individual variations in response to them, but with their prophylactic use, exercise-induced asthma can be prevented in 90% of patients.[2] Athletes with asthma who are taking antiasthma drugs and who are planning to compete in world class competitions are advised to have their physicians provide documentation well in advance to the United States Olympic Committee for drug use clearance.[6]

MANAGING ALLERGIC RHINITIS AND RESPIRATORY CONGESTION IN THE ATHLETE

Many athletes may experience transient breathing problems due to allergic rhinitis (hay fever), upper respiratory viral infections (the common cold), and sinusitis; a decrease in physical performance and endurance may result from these maladies. Treatment of the symptoms of nasal and respiratory congestion may consist of topical or systemic medications. Several classes of drugs are available for symptomatic treatment and they include H_1-antagonist antihistamines, sympathomimetic vasoconstrictor decongestants, cromolyn sodium, aerosolized glucocorticosteroids, nonopiate analgesics, and opiate antitussives (e.g., cough suppressants). International Olympic Committee (IOC) rules ban the use of any sympathomimetic decongestants, opioid analgesics, and opioid antitussives. Although antihistamines are effective in alleviating the symptoms of hay fever or the common cold, side effects such as drowsiness, decreased motor coordination, and anticholinergic-induced impairment of sweating may interfere with an athlete's performance. A recently approved antihistamine, terfenadine, causes less drowsiness than the traditional H_1-antihistamines[34]; this effect, along with the drug's action on motor coordination, should be studied further in athletes. If it shows clear advantage with less anticholinergic, sedative, and motor coordination side effects in this patient population, it would be the antihistamine of choice in athletes. Data to support this are lacking at this time. Sympathomimetic vasoconstriction decongestants have the advantages of not causing drowsiness and of being effectively administered by both the topical and systemic routes. They act by causing vasoconstriction in the mucous membranes of the nasal passages. Chronic frequent topical application of these agents can result in a "vicious cycle" type of rebound nasal congestion called rhinitis medicamentosum. Systemic administration of these drugs can result in increased heart rate, increased blood pressure, and increased blood glucose levels in susceptible individuals and is not allowed by the IOC. Cromolyn sodium nasal spray is effective in preventing allergy-based hay fever, but has no place in the treatment of the common cold. It is thought to work by several mechanisms to stabilize the membrane of the mast cell, thus preventing the release of histamine and other chemical mediators and their resultant symptoms. The newer aerosolized steroids, such as beclomethasone and flunisolide, are also effective in treating hay fever; they have the advantage of not being systemically absorbed.

Respiratory symptoms such as cough in the athlete may be alleviated by opiate analgesic antitussives (for example, codeine and hydrocodone). Opiates are quite effective in suppressing a cough by their action on the central nervous system cough center in the medulla. They have many side effects, but those noteworthy in the athlete include possible respiratory depression, nausea, drowsiness, light-headedness, and the potential for physical dependence. Nonopiate antitussives include dextromethorphan (common in many nonprescription cough preparations) and diphenhydramine (an antihistamine). Dextromethorphan in regular doses has few side effects, although drowsiness and nausea may occur. Diphenhydramine shares the same side effects as the other antihistamines outlined above. Productive and purulent coughs should not be supressed; dry hacking coughs may be safely supressed. It is important to remember that water and proper hydration can act as an excellent expectorant, aiding in proper mucosal physiology. Because of the widespread availability of nonprescription cough and cold preparations, many athletes do not consider them to be potent drugs; this is a misconception and their use should be reported to athletic trainers and team physicians, so that monitoring for potential adverse effects may occur. Dextromethorphan is not banned by the IOC and may be used as an antitussive by competing athletes.

MANAGING MOTION SICKNESS IN THE ATHLETE

Motion sickness is caused when visual and vestibular stimuli are imbalanced, such as when the head rotates in two axes simultaneously.[27] Drugs that are effective in preventing and controlling the nausea and vomiting associated with motion sickness are the antihistamines, scopolamine, and some phenothiazines. They are believed to work by suppressing the chemoreceptor trigger zone in the brain. Antihistamines commonly used in this disorder are dimenhydrinate, cyclizine, and meclizine. Dimenhydrinate (Dramamine) doses for adults are 50 to 100 mg, two to four times per day. Cyclizine (Marezine) doses are 50 mg up to four times per day. Meclizine (Antivert, Bonine) is longer acting and is administered in doses of 25 to 50 mg once a day. The most common side effect of these drugs is sedation. Scopolamine, available by prescription only, is effective and is available as an adhesive patch that is applied to the skin once every three days. It has strong anticholinergic side effects, such as dry mouth, impaired sweating, blurred vision, and constipation. Prochlorperazine is the phenothiazine that is commonly used for nausea and vomiting. Some of its side effects include extrapyramidal reactions, drowsiness, and anticholinergic effects. The athlete with the nausea and vomiting of motion sickness should be assessed closely, and such causes as a blow to the head, sinusitis, or influenza should be ruled out before participation in competition is allowed. Side effects of any of the above mentioned antiemetic drugs may interfere with the fine-motor coordination, sweating, vision, or concentration needed during participation in many sports.

TREATING NOCTURNAL LEG MUSCLE CRAMPS

Nocturnal cramps affect the calf muscles of the leg or occur in the foot and have no known cause. They may be associated with strenuous exercise or fatigue, and may occur in all age groups; they are rarely associated with any underlying pathology.[9] Common modalities of treatment include massage and stretching of the affected limb and muscle groups, and prophylactic administration of diphenhydramine (Benadryl), 25 to 50 mg, or quinine sulfate, 300 mg at bedtime.

Proof of efficacy of these drugs in a healthy population is difficult to find, although a double-blind, crossover study was done in healthy elderly patients comparing quinine sulfate to placebo. In this study, 300 mg of quinine was found to be significantly superior to placebo in decreasing the number, severity, and duration of nocturnal cramps.[18] Extrapolating these results to healthy young athletes is difficult, however, because of the increased age and the small number of patients studied. Quinine is believed to work in nocturnal cramps because it increases the skeletal muscle refractory period, and allows less skeletal muscle responses to occur after repeated nerve stimulation.[18] Massage and stretching of the affected muscle groups are probably the treatment of choice for nocturnal cramps in healthy athletes, but dehydration, total body water deficit due to sweating, and incorrectly fitted athletic shoes must be assessed and corrected in this population. The use of drugs to treat leg and foot cramps should not be commonly necessary in the healthy athlete.

THE USE OF ANABOLIC STEROIDS IN ATHLETES

The use of anabolic steroids has been estimated to be from 90% to 100% in national and international male competitors in bodybuilding, weight lifting, and shot put, hammer, discus, and javelin throwing.[21] In light of the bans against the use of these drugs by the International Olympic Committee, such widespread use of anabolic steroids is sobering. It is of particular concern also that with such an example being set for younger athletes, they may accept anabolic steroid usage as the norm and adopt its use without being informed of the dangers inherent in such abusive practices. Those who work closely with athletes should understand the myriad adverse effects of the anabolic steroids, and should make every effort to educate athletes about these effects and strongly discourage their use. Supplies of the drugs are obtained most commonly by diversion from normal drug distribution paths, so that those working closely with athletes must be cognizant of the need to question the athlete to ascertain previously unreported anabolic steroid usage.

Although the side effects of these drugs are well described, scientific evidence for their efficacy in increasing strength is controversial. Lamb, in an excellent review of anabolic steroids,[21] described common regimens of injectable and oral steroids being used at 10 to 40 times normal therapeutic doses. Regimens include combining high doses of both dosage forms for weeks to months before a competition and quickly tapering the drugs in the weeks immediately prior to competition to circumvent detection through drug testing. Subjective claims of efficacy by athletes include increased muscle mass, increased muscle strength, and aggressiveness; all of these effects, if true, could lead to more efficient training and better performance in competitions. Scientific studies, which have used significantly lower doses than those currently used by athletes, have shown an average weight gain of about 5 lb in those subjects studied. Studies of muscle strength are divided equally as to whether or not significant improvement has occurred. Aerobic work capacity has not been shown to improve with anabolic steroid use.[21]

Anabolic steroids can cause serious, varied, and potentially irreversible side effects. Of particular note to those working with young athletes is premature and permanent closure of the epiphyses in long bones.[10] Mental changes attributed to steroid use include increased aggressiveness, mood changes, and, rarely, psychosis. Sexual changes in men include decreased libido, gynecomastia, testicular atrophy, suppression of natural testosterone levels, and decreased spermatogenesis. Irreversible virilization can occur in women taking anabolic steroids. Acne and oily skin occur commonly; elevations of hepatic enzyme levels and, rarely, hepatic cancer have been reported with use of these drugs. Fluid retention can occur, which may lead to polydrug abuse, when diuretics are taken to counteract this effect.[16] Long-term effects on the cardiovascular system have not been reported but could be expected, theoretically.

The question of risk vs. benefit with this class of drugs may be clouded by the athlete's desire to win. Questions of efficacy, safety, and ethics are also overshadowed by this, as evidenced by the widespread use and abuse of the anabolic steroids. One can only hope that education and guidance of the next generation of athletes will prepare them to learn from their predecessors' mistakes and allow them to decline the unnecessary use of this potentially dangerous class of drugs.

ACKNOWLEDGMENTS

The author wishes to acknowledge the assistance and contributions of Ms. Betsy Torg and Mr. Joe Vegso in the preparation of this manuscript.

REFERENCES

1. Anderson LA, Gatzsche PC: Naproxen and aspirin in acute musculoskeletal disorders: A double blind, parallel study in patients with sports injuries. *Pharmotherapeutica* 1984; 3:531–537.

2. Anderson SD: Drugs affecting the respiratory system with particular reference to asthma. *Med Sci Sports* 1981; 13:259–265.

3. Beaver WT: Aspirin and acetaminophen as constituents of analgesic combinations. *Arch Intern Med* 1981; 141:293–300.

4. Bierman CW: A comparison of late reactions to antigen and exercise. *J Allergy Clin Immunol* 1984; 73:657.

5. Brogden RN, et al: Naproxen up to date: A review of its pharmacological properties and therapeutic efficacy and use in rheumatic diseases and pain states. *Drugs* 1979; 18:266.

6. Clarke KS: Sports medicine and drug control programs of the U.S. Olympic Committee. *J Allergy Clin Immunol* 1984; 73:740–744.

7. Clancy WC: Exercise induced asthma. *Am J Sports Med* 1981; 9(3):194–196.

8. Cooper SA: Five studies on ibuprofen for postsurgical dental pain. *Am J Med* 1984; 77:70–77.

9. Cutler P: Queries and minor notes: Then and now: Cramps in the legs and feet. *JAMA* 1984; 252:98.

10. Drugs in the olympics. *Med Letter* 1984; 26:66.

11. Elenbaas JK: Centrally acting skeletal muscle relaxants. *Am J Hosp Pharm* 1980; 37:1313–1323.

12. Filho JL: Multicenter study of piroxicam in the treatment of acute musculoskeletal diseases among 3,011 patients. *Eur J Rheumatol Inflamm* 1983; 6:119.

13. Foley KM: The treatment of cancer pain. *N Engl J Med* 1985; 313:84–85.

14. Fox S: Icing and heating: Which and when in management of sports injury. *Med News Int Rep* 1985; 9:13.

15. Godfrey S: Introduction to symposium on special problems and management of allergic athletes. *J Allergy Clin Immunol* 1984; 73:630–632.

16. Hill J, et al: The athletic polydrug abuse phenomenon. *Am J Sports Med* 1983; 11(4):269–271.

17. Hocutt JE, et al: Cryotherapy in ankle sprains. *Am J Sports Med* 1982; 10(5):318.

18. Jones K, Castleden CM: A double-blind comparison of quinine sulfate and placebo in muscle cramps. *Age Aging* 1983; 12:155–158.

19. Katz RM: Rhinitis in the athlete. *J Allergy Clin Immunol* 1984; 73:708–711.

20. Konig P: The use of cromolyn in the management of hyperactive airways and exercise. *J Allergy Clin Immunol* 1984; 73:686.

21. Lamb DR: Anabolic steroids in athletics: How well do they work and how dangerous are they? *Am J Sports Med* 1984; 12(1):31–38.

22. Lane HW, et al: Effect of physical activity on human potassium metabolism in a hot and humid environment. *Am J Clin Nutrition* 1978; 31:838–843.

23. Levy G: Comparative pharmacokinetics of aspirin and acetaminophen. *Arch Intern Med* 1981; 141:279–281.

24. Mehlisch DR: Review of the comparative analgesic efficacy of salicylates, acetaminophen and pyrazolones. *Am J Med* 1983; 75:47–52.

25. Muckle DS: Comparative study of ibuprofen and aspirin in soft tissue injuries. *Rheumatol Rehabil* 1974; 13:141–147.

26. Murphy RJ: Heat illness in the athlete. *Am J Sports Med* 1984; 12(4):258–261.

27. Oderda GM, West S: Emetic and antiemetic products, in *Handbook of Nonprescription Drugs*, ed 7. Washington, DC, American Pharmaceutical Association, 1982, pp 100–101.

28. Reynolds RC, Floetz P, Thielke TS: Comparative analysis of drug distribution costs for controlled versus noncontrolled oral analgesics. *Am J Hosp Pharm* 1984; 41:1558–1563.

29. Santilli G, et al: Comparative study with piroxican and ibuprofen versus placebo in the supportive treatment of minor sports injuries. *J Int Med Res* 1980; 8:265–269.

30. Settipane GA: Adverse reactions to aspirin and related drugs. *Arch Intern Med* 1981; 141:328–332.
31. Sly M: Exercise induced asthma. *South Med J* 1978; 71:111–117.
32. Sly RM: Beta adrenergic drugs in the management of asthma in athletes. *J Allergy Clin Immunol* 1984; 73:680–685.
33. Smith NJ: The prevention of heat disorders in sports. *AJDC* 1984; 138:786–790.
34. Sorkin EM, Heel RC: Terfenadine: A review of its pharmacodynamic properties and therapeutic efficacy. *Drugs* 1985; 29:35–36.
35. Szczeklik A: Antipyretic analgesics and the allergic patient. *Am J Med* 1983; 75:82–84.
36. Wallenstein SL, et al: Relative analgesic potency of oral zomepirac and intramuscular morphine in cancer patients with postoperative pain. *J Clin Pharmacol* 1980; 20:250–258.
37. Yackzan L, Adams C, Francis KT: The effects of ice massage on delayed muscle soreness. *Am J Sports Med* 1984; 12(2):160.
38. Zanecosky A: Salt, potassium, and electrolyte drinks. *University of Pennsylvania Sports Med Newsletter* 1984; 1:1–2.

Index